CALISTHENICS

Complete Step by Step Workout Guide to Build Strength

(Accelerated Beginner's Guide to Calisthenics and Strength)

Carolyn Thompson

Published By Darby Connor

Carolyn Thompson

All Rights Reserved

Calisthenics: Complete Step by Step Workout Guide to Build Strength (Accelerated Beginner's Guide to Calisthenics and Strength)

ISBN 978-1-77485-287-3

Legal & Disclaimer

The information contained in this book is not designed to replace or take the place of any form of medicine or professional medical advice. The information in this book has been provided for educational and entertainment purposes only.

The information contained in this book has been compiled from sources deemed reliable, and it is accurate to the best of the Author's knowledge; however, the Author cannot guarantee its accuracy and validity and cannot be held liable for any errors or omissions. Changes are periodically made to this book. You must consult your doctor or get professional medical advice before using any of the suggested remedies, techniques, or information in this book.

TABLE OF CONTENTS

Introduction

Being able to have a healthy body and the right amount of fat requires a lot of dedication and hard work and this is something that no one will argue with. However, what we cannot dispute but is that to achieve that toned and attractive body, you have to put in many hours in the gym hitting weights like your life was on the line.

In a world in which, to live people have to be working a 9-5 job, and sometimes even multiple jobs, not to mention the long hours we are In the car as well as stuck in traffic jams. average person is losing 42 hours of their time each year due to traffic congestion. Therefore, finding time to exercise may not be possible. Do you think that just because you are unable to go for a workout, that you have to let the fat build up and your muscles deteriorate? Absolutely not!

Strength training is a great method to shape your body and plan some time for gym workouts within your routine even if you can't get in the gym there's other exercises you can try to get the benefits of strengthening without the need to visit the gym. Calisthenics is one of these types of exercise.

What exactly are calisthenics, and how can you begin with the exercise? This is the aim of this article to teach you how you can use calisthenics to build a body that you're proud of.

Chapter 1: Calisthenics 101

Calisthenics, as with other fitness programs is a type of exercise that helps in the improvement of one's physical strength however unlike other types of programs it focuses on training the body's weight and is not dependent on gym equipment. Because there are various types of exercise with identical concepts, this definition of the specific workout could be somewhat ambiguous and is able to be generalized easily. In a handful of cases, particularly for those who are new to the sport, it does not differ from other exercise routine, but it can be.

Calisthenics

Like we said, calisthenics is a kind of exercise that originates directly from Greek terms kalos (meaning beauty) and sthenos (meaning strength). It is often thought to be akin to other type of workout. By those who don't grasp the concept, and view it as a routine that is related to gymnastics and is misinterpreted as a type of yoga.

The primary thing that distinguishes calisthenics is its focus solely on body weight training and weight conditioning. Its goal is to provide you with greater control over the body and body actions. After a few weeks the aim is to help you become more coordinated, agile and more flexible.

Furthermore, a calisthenics session is possible to do at practically any place, whether it's at home or at the office it is possible to exercise whenever you like. If you have enough space for your preferred exercises, you're ready to go. Since exercise equipment isn't required, you'll be able to go about your daily routine with ease.

Calisthenics for both men and Women

One of the benefits for calisthenics exercise is the fact that nearly everyone can add it into their fitness routine that is suitable for both women. Men, in particular, are enthralled by the possibility to release excess energy and helping their health Some choose to do more intense exercise routines.

However exercising in calisthenics is beneficial for women too. There are exceptions however certain women are more suited to moderate exercise; they typically opt for exercises that don't require them to sweat a lot. In addition this particular type of weight training for the body is believed to promote healthy pregnancy. As studies have shown, it combats gestational diabetes and increases the fitness of the lungs and heart rate.

Things to Take into Account

While it comes with a lot of benefits however, it can only benefit you by your participation. It demands consistency and dedication. If you stop from your training, be sure you return soon to them and avoid long breaks. Rememberthat 3-4 days of not exercising could impede your improvement. A workout every day (that can be completed in about an half an hour, or even less) is ideal, however when this isn't possible only a few times can be sufficient.

Things to Consider:

Personal fitness goals in training

What's your ultimate objective in starting an exercise program that includes calisthenics? Once you've figured that out, you're able to start your workouts. Once you have figured out your motivation it will be easier to feel enthusiastic to begin the exercises.

Schedule

If you're contemplating implementing the calisthenics routine take your time and put your availability into the equation. Go through your schedule and decide if you have the time to train often. Since the majority of calisthenics exercises can be completed in any vacant space It's easy to adjust your schedule to add a few minutes for the specific physical exercise.

The Five Advantages to Calisthenics

A common benefit of a calisthenics workout is its general fitness as well as its capacity to provide great neural adaption and strengthening of your base, build your strength and help you overcome a variety of physiological difficulties. While it isn't difficult to achieve but it will improve your overall well-being.

It is a fact that calisthenics training exercises can also be used to aid in reaching almost any fitness goal is widely acknowledged. If you want bigger muscle mass or desire to be a beast of strength, exercise routines for weight training could aid you. As long as you select the right exercises, you'll be happy with your results within a month of time.

Additionally, by selecting carefully selected calisthenics exercises, you can take a few minutes of your time for exercises, and you'll notice an improvement in your overall performance. Furthermore, since the range of activities is straightforward, you'll not be exhausted from just the idea of a vigorous workout.

The benefits are:

1. Improved breathing

If you're suffering from respiratory illnesses regularly, calisthenics training sessions are suggested. For a suggestion, consider making sure that your workouts focus on building your spine or fixing your posture.

2. More energy

If you're exhausted every single day exercising in calisthenics could be the best option for you. They trigger certain body cells which can increase your strength and flexibility. If you're experiencing issues with your sexuality It could be time to hop on the into calisthenics.

3. Better mental awareness

According to researchers at the University of Southwestern Texas, calisthenics is the preferred choice for people who require assistance with their mental health

Research has proven that they're less stressful for our nervous systems. The body-training workouts provide there are a myriad positive mental benefits can be derived such as improved sleep, higher concentration levels, enhanced memory, an improved outlook on life (i.e. you are more optimistic) and lower level of stress and fatigue.

4. Joint pain relief

In comparison to any other exercise calisthenics exercises, which are an exercise that is based on exercise that involves body weight are believed to be gentler for joints. This is because the resistance you'll encounter is your own body weight. If you're struggling with issues such as tendonitis, arthritis as well as other joint problems following regular calisthenics workouts is advised.

5. Weight loss

Calisthenics can be a more secure alternative to taking weight loss medication. The results may not be as quick, however they are not at any risk.

Additional Reasons to Consider the Use of an Calisthenics Workout Routine

Take a look at famous personalities like Arthur Saxon, John Grimek as well as Sig Klein. They all have an beautiful bodies because of their use of a calisthenics exercise routine. Not only did they adopt the great bodyweight exercise routine, but they also spent several months or even years to learn the specific method; and with the results, you can see that they weren't wrong by doing it.

Other motives:

It can be done anyplace.

It is affordable and does not need equipment for exercise

Menopausal mood swings are a common cause.

It's not hard to incorporate

Facilitates faster recovery from certain diseases.

Chapter 2: The 6 Types Of Calisthenic Exercises

Every calisthenic workout should be broken down into six patterns of functional movement.

This is the only kind of exercise that you should do to build your muscles, strengthen and tone.

It also encompasses...

1. Exercises for the upper body:

Exercises for upper body compression will strengthen the pressing muscles of your upper body.

These muscles comprise

The chest,

the front shoulder,

The medial shoulders

and the strong and powerful triceps.

They are crucial as they teach you how to keep a steady shoulder position when pushing things away.

A pressing on the upper part of the body could be further divided into a vertical and horizontal pressing. vertical pressing.

More details on this to come...

#No. 2 . Upper body pull exercises to strengthen the body.

Exercises for the upper back work the muscles in your back to lift the objects up on you.

These muscles comprise

the back shoulder,

the rhombuses

the trapezius

The lats

and the and the

They are essential as they aid in correcting any imbalances in your muscles shoulders and help you develop the ability to lift yourself from the ground or onto an edge.

A pull of the upper part of your body could be split into a horizontal and vertical pull.

More on this in the near future...

#3 Knee Flex Exercises:

Exercises that bend your knees work the muscles that permit you to squat before being able return to doing squats.

These muscles comprise

the quadriceps muscles,

the adductors

the many other muscles of the hip

and the buttocks

They are essential as they improve the ability of squatting to be in the correct posture. Before the invention of toilets we used squats to get rid of ourselves.

Four One-Legged Exercises:

One-legged exercises help you learn to maintain your balance with each foot. If you haven't noticed it before, it's time to do it now. You're spending the majority of your time on one leg.

These exercises will build

the quadriceps

the adductors

the musculature's core

and all those smaller stabilizing muscles are usually not stimulated in bilateral exercises.

They are essential as they help improve your balance and coordination as well as correcting any imbalances among your legs.

#No. 5 hip extension exercises:

The exercises for hip extension train the muscles of the back chain, which can aid in stretching and bending your hips.

These muscles comprise

the muscles of the hamstrings

the buttocks,

The lower and upper back.

The importance of these exercises is that they help you learn the proper hip flexion, which can lessen the chance of back injuries in the lower back.

Finally, we are left with...

#6 Stabilizing core exercises:

In case you didn't realize it already: sit-ups or crunches are not the most effective method to strengthen those abdominal muscles. It's not the ideal method of training your abdominal muscles.

You should instead develop the core stabilization. This means the ability to hold back any movement during a load.

An instance of a core stabilization workout is the plank, and the various variations of it.

In this article, we will concentrate on these fundamental 6 motion patterns. These are the movements that should be the norm for 99% all of humanity.

Now having covered the essentials, let's move on to the exciting part.

In the next chapter the complete list of gymnastic activities by body part and degree of difficulty is reviewed.

Continue reading...

Chapter 3: The Routines

Routine #1 Basic Strength

This is the first exercise that is most straightforward and simple, but it's still a bit challenging, so don't be discouraged in the least If yours is what you select for the first time. That's actually the entire purpose! This workout will help you get moving and will begin to target the major muscle groups that calisthenics are all about .

With no breaks between Here are the steps:

8 reps: Extensive toe taps

10 reps: Push-ups with an elevated bar.

1o reps: Leg raises

15, reps: Step Ups

10 reps: Bench dips

Twenty reps Squats

Routine #2: Cardio Quick-Start

This second exercise is a bit more difficult and includes strength-based exercises that can get your heart pumping to provide a full-body workout.

10 reps: Bench dips

50 reps: Crunches

Ten reps Burpees

25, reps: Squat Jacks

10 repetitions 10 reps: Jump rope

20 reps 20 reps: Push-ups

Routine #3: 1-Cycle Burn

This workout is tough enough that it's only necessary to do it once! Here are the steps...

30-reps Jump Squats

30-reps Squat Jacks

Repetition of 15: Burpees

15 reps: Bench dips

15 reps: Jumping lunges

10 reps 10 reps: Push-ups

4-Cycle Routine

This is a great third step for the more experienced person or those seeking a true test. Here are the stepsto follow:

Five reps Burpees

50 reps 50 reps: Push-ups

25 reps for Jump Squats: 25 reps

15 reps 15 reps

15 reps: Leg raises

10 reps 10 reps

Repeat this two times with 3 minutes of rest between cycles.

Route #5 3Cycle Circuit

The circuit should be repeated three times as long as you can handle it. If you're committed to this circuit simply because you enjoy the movements then you should begin to do this circuit only once this morning, and then repeat it twice when you are ready. Don't overdo it or you'll end up injured and frustrated. Be patient and you'll make it!

Ten reps Burpees

10 reps: Bench dips

15 reps: Jumping lunges

15 reps Squats jumps

20 repetitions: Squat Jacks

30 reps 30 reps: Push-ups

Pause between circuits as required.

Route #6: The Ultimate Circuit

This exercise can be done at least three times in succession with no break between. The pattern follows a formula that is easy to pick up:

30 repetitions 30 reps: Jump Squats

20 reps 20 reps: Push-ups

10 reps: Jumping Lunges

Ten reps Burpees

20 repetitions: Leg Flutters

30-reps Squat Jacks

Are you taking a break?

It's good to rest But so is challenging yourself. It's possible to need 10 15 or 30 seconds of take a break between your moves, particularly during your third or second cycle. If you're required to rest for three to five minutes between workouts, do it. Be careful not to drink excessive amounts of water prior to and during the workout in order to not feel sick, but afterward, make sure you drink plenty of water.

If you decide to take a break it doesn't mean you lie on the mat or sit down. Move from between feet and remain alert to avoid throwing off your body's pulse. Continue to move, but do it at a gentle pace while waiting for the next step to start.

Advanced Modifications

There is an endless number of sophisticated modifications to all of these moves. Here are a few of the most well-known:

The push-up is complicated by doing it with one hand or by supporting yourself using your legs not touching the ground , but lifted from the floor.

Burpees may be made more challenging by a variety of methods. When you return to your plank position, lower into a pushup, before getting your feet back up and standing to complete an squat leap.

Leg flapping can be made challenging by finding that sweet place of struggle. Stretch your legs straight in the air , then slowly lower them toward the ground until you feel the pain in your abdominal muscles. This is the ideal height to be kicking at.

"With Control"

A popular phrases you'll hear during your exercise is"with the control". What exactly does it mean to accomplish something"with in control"? In essence, it means that you're not letting momentum or gravity dictate your actions, and you're in total control of the action. This usually means that you're moving slow. In terms of fitness it is best to do it slowly!

Proper Form

If you're performing one of these exercises it is important to ensure you're performing the move with the correct technique. If you're not properly formed, it's difficult to perform the move and can make your exercise ineffective and could result in injury in your own body. Always be sure to check your own form as you do your exercise routine.

One of the biggest errors people make when exercising is not keeping their lower backs pressed against the mat when doing ab movements. This can cause serious injury to the lower back, therefore it is essential to work your abs as well as suck your belly button into ensure your lower back remains flat onto the mat. If you're struggling assistance, put your hands on your tailbone to assist in pressing your back to the floor.

Engaging Your Body

Engaging your body during your workout will automatically improve your fitness posture regardless of what you're working on. Engage your abs that means you've got your belly button engaged instead of being relaxing and lazy. When you engage your body in this way, in this way, you'll sit up more upright and feel more stable and stronger naturally. Make sure to keep this in mind during your training.

One of the most efficient methods of ensuring you're in the proper posture is to examine yourself each time you take a break between exercises or cycles. Try to pay attention to your posture as you wait for your next movement to start.

Breathing

Breathing is among the most essential factors in a successful exercise and staying fit. In the moment, put your hands on your stomach and breathe in. If your belly seemed to expand like the majority of people feel, then you must work on your breathing. As you breathe in, it's not difficult to let your belly and chest expand. However, it's best to start breathing in a way that your sides are puffing out instead.

If you attempt to breathe out towards from the sides, you'll find that you naturally contract your abs to accomplish this. This means that you only need to focus on one thing: whether you keep your abs in a state of engagement or keep your breathing towards the side while you exercise to achieve both! Isn't that going to make your workout simpler?

When you breathe it is important to be paying attention to the way you breathe. In the ideal scenario, you'll breathe through your nose, and exhale through your mouth during your work out. This breathing technique allows you to get enough air in your lungs, while helping keep the heart in good shape and supple with oxygen.

Final Precautions

I hope that you will enjoy the routines, regardless of how you decide to tackle them. Once you've started ensure that you take it slow initially. It's a lot of fun to put caution to the wind and start moving forward whenever you're full of determination however, exhausting yourself or injuring yourself on day one will not make it very far.

Slow down, take your time and adjust your pace according to your needs. This will keep your body in a constant state of alert and keep pushing toward your target. Do not stop once you've started!

Chapter 4: Calisthenics Training:

Guide to Getting Started Guide

Be aware that using the gross muscles to exercise your body isn't easy. For example, if you are extremely overweight, performing one pull-up--let alone many in succession--will not be simple. Due to this, it is essential to, in the event that you are overweight, choose a diet that encourages weight reduction. To achieve this, when you participate in the workouts we'll be discussing in the next sections of the book think about taking a clean eating diet like that of the FitMole diet or Paleo diet. These diets ensure that when you follow the exercises we'll talk about later, you'll notice a significant weight loss.

Once we've got the food part gone Let's discuss another aspect that is equally important. If you're new to calisthenics you may be asking yourself questions like:

"Which exercises should be part of my exercise routine every day?"

"How do I know the amount of training, how often should I plan the training?"

"How numerous repetitions can I perform in each workout?"

"What do you think about resting between reps? How do you think it should be?"

Undoubtedly, not having the answers may cause your program to be in limbo, which could cause you to lose motivation. In this section of the guide, you'll find all the details you require to start calisthenics and not feel overwhelmed.

Getting Started

The first thing to think about is your degree of physical fitness.

The majority of calisthenics-related programs can be classified into three categories three categories: intermediate, beginner, and advanced. Compare these levels to your fitness level, and then determine which level you'd like to start at. If you're not fit, begin with the very first step: the beginner stage. If you're fit, you could begin at an intermediate level and, if you are fit, begin at the advanced level. The benefit of calisthenics is that, even if you start at the simplest level, as your abilities improve and you gain strength you can progress to intermediate, and eventually advanced.

To get there, however, you must begin, which is the purpose of this section to aid you in doing. The information we'll cover here will be geared towards the total beginner

Step 1: Determine Your Start Point and define your goals

Do not be one of the novices who when getting to a point, don't spend the time to evaluate their initial point of departure. If you don't you're harming yourself because when you don't have a clear idea of where you are starting and your objectives, selecting which exercises and exercises to do can be a bit difficult.

For instance, if you follow an exercise routine for calisthenics which requires you to perform an chin or push up but you can't do eitherof these, then you won't reap benefits from the exercise routine. In addition you must also be able to master the basic body weight exercises before you begin implementing the exercises we will be discussing in the later sections of this book.

In the same vein of thinking, your goals for training will determine the type of exercises you include in your schedule, particularly because there are many different types of exercises. What is this and what can you do? Think about the following:

For Weight Loss

If you're looking to shed some weight, no matter which calisthenics routine you decide to do, ensure that your time between sets is not too long. The aim is to raise your heart rate so that you will burn more calories and, in turn, lose weight. If you incorporate longer periods of rest your heart rate will decline, which means lower fat loss.

For Muscle strength and gains in mass

If your aim is to build muscle and increase your strength, plan longer intervals between sets to maximize recovery of your muscles and continue exercising at your desired intensities. Also you must focus on your posture and pay attention to your connection between mind and muscle so that you can focus your energy.

To provide Endurance and Stamina

If your goal is to increase stamina and endurance, try the bodyweight exercise that includes intense exercises and aerobic exercise. While this can help improve your endurance, it'll make little difference in helping you increase muscles (however it will help shape the muscles). As you will see that determining your goals will aid you in determining where to begin.

Step 2: Decide the amount of time you can devote to working out

How much time you are able to put into training will determine when you'll see any improvements. Once you've started exercising, you need to do so every 3-4 days for 30-60 minutes according to your fitness level and the calisthenics workout program you're adhering to.

Exercise for 3-4 days each week until you progress into the intermediate or expert level. You can then decide how long you will need to exercise each week to reach your objectives.

Step 3. Determine the Needed Equipment

As mentioned earlier, even though calisthenics workouts are bodyweight exercises which do not need gym equipment. However, equipment like a pull up bar or ab wheel or gymnast rings can provide an exciting twist to your workouts and result in better outcomes. Therefore, it is important to know what equipment you have in your possession and then figure out the items you require and how you can afford to do in order to achieve this. As we have seen earlier, the majority of these products don't cost much , and If you can't purchase the most basic equipment, you could come up with your own ideas.

Once we have the basic rules in place Let us define and then talk about the essential calisthenics exercises that are ideal for novices:

Chapter 5: Hints and Tricks for Beginners to Avoid Making Mistakes

How to make the right Fortschritt

In the beginning, calisthenics comes from Greek words meaning the beauty of and strength. It is essentially movements, flexibility techniques, the ability to withstand the elements. It's not as easy like adding weights onto bars.

Your body's weight is enough to begin. If you're working out in a gym or with a pull-up bar everything will help your body build muscles as time passes. However, calisthenics requires you understand your body's capabilities and your own to increase the quality of your workout.

Selecting The Best Exercise

There are a variety of exercises that are available to those who are just beginning. A few of the fundamental and fundamental exercises in calisthenics include push-ups, dips, push-ups in squats, abdominal exercises. If you are doing any kind of training, it's important to identify the areas of your body you wish to target.

Certain exercises can assist you to strengthen your legs and abs, for instance for example, leg raises, or those which help to develop muscles on the top of your part of your body such as with abs. It is advised to start with the basics as you'll become accustomed to it. Push-ups and push-ups for instance, can be the base for more difficult exercises. Therefore, it is crucial to grasp a solid understanding of the fundamentals.

You can go from the Easy to Hard

If you begin working out, you'll think that you can accomplish numerous things. Being a superhero isn't a bad thing in and of itself. However, it is crucial to maintain some self-control limits and be patient and take the steps one at a time in the exercise routine. This means you should begin with simple exercises to prepare yourself for more complex and difficult exercises. If you do this you'll be able to stay safe from injury and make sure that you are willing to explore more techniques, variations and postures.

How to get the right posture

The posture is crucial when performing calisthenics, since it can affect the effectiveness of the exercise. Making sure that your body (core arm, shoulders, as well as your legs) is properly aligned for a successful performance of the exercises. Many people make mistakes by doing calisthenics in the wrong manner or not being able to control the movements of exercises and techniques.

The training for calisthenics requires patience for your body to adapt and produce tangible outcomes. It is therefore essential to know how to properly exercise from the beginning, rather than be astonished by the prospect of doing intense repetitions in the beginning.

Safety Caution

Before beginning calisthenics, it is crucial to begin with basic exercises such as the push-ups and more to help the body get used with the workout routine. It is only then that it is recommended to move on to more strenuous exercises.

A thing to keep in mind is the strain that is put on joints while exercising. It is crucial to keep in mind that your tendons and ligaments are more active during exercise, as opposed to lifting weights in the gym. The reason for this is the movement performed in calisthenics exercises.

Make sure you rest correctly when putting your wrists and shoulders, for instance, when you exert a lot of exertion, so that you avoid serious injuries. You should also allow yourself the time to heal.

If you are feeling that you're overweight, it might be beneficial to follow a nutritious diet to lose weight prior to taking up calisthenics. Certain cardio exercises could be beneficial, should they be needed.

A few pounds off can make you more able to do your training and build up muscle.

Rest, Respiration, And Recovery

Make sure you breathe through every exercise. This will build your strength and prevent you from dying. Inhale for the initial part of the exercise (concentric movement upwards) and exhale to complete the second part (eccentric movement downwards). You are free to add intervals between workouts, and between sets. If you're unable to complete a particular workout you can try a simpler variation and work up from there.

Chapter 6: The Bodyweight Progression

So , we've talked about some of the most difficult moves, and also the basics of moves. Let's look at how we can link them!

What exactly is Bodyweight Progression?

In starting your workout typically, you will use less difficult exercises or lighter weights. However, when you get "used" to the exercises or weights and you get accustomed to them, you can make them somewhat more difficult by adding weights or onto more challenging exercises. This is known as progress.

It is common for people to use progression to achieve their goals since getting into the most difficult exercise that you could find might not be feasible at your current level of fitness. If, for instance, you're a novice cyclist, would you choose to go right to "Le Tour of France"? Absolutely not. At the very least, you should begin working towards a minimum 10-mile run at first. The same applies to bodyweight and weight progression.

Bodyweight progression occurs used in the same technique for calisthenics. For this to be done in calisthenics you'll need to begin with simple moves before progressing to more challenging ones. In other words, for instance you might not be able to perform exercises for muscle on the first day of your visit to the gym. It is important to build your muscle before going for this one.

One way to use the bodyweight to progress to the stage of a muscle-up is to learn how to pull-up before you master it. Begin with a more comfortable grip for you is the most effective method to learn how to pull-up. Once you've got pulled-ups you are comfortable with it is time to practice your dips. A dip occurs where you start on the bar and then dive into it. You can master them by tripping dips with your fist on the lower surfaces. In this way, you do not have to stand over the bar.

Now that you know what you can do with the dip and pull-up and dip, you can try the change from a pull-up into a dip, and the reverse. It is the second part of the muscle-up. you'll need to learn how to climb up onto the bar and then back down without falling and injury to yourself. Experts advise being strong when transitioning from dips to pull-ups.

When you've got all three parts learned and you're confident in your ability to piece them all together, go for it! You're now capable of doing the exercise! This could take a few weeks to master the desired results, and could require months. You must be perseverant and hardworking.

The best way to do this is to break down more difficult moves into comparable (or, in this instance the same, simple movements that you can try to help you reach your goals.

Why should I use Progression?

Why not just jump right into the more challenging move? It is possible to practice this move until you master the technique isn't it? Yes. You can try it but it's not a success. It may take some time for you to notice improvement.

Why not just forget about being disappointed and get back to work? Training is the best way to ensure that you'll get stronger in more than just one area of your body. This is contrary to the notion that you'll only become stronger (at an incredibly slower rate, if even) within the one area which you're working on.

For instance, you would like to be able to perform the 90 degree push-up. This happens when your body is suspended in position in the air with an angle, and you perform a higher. If you are unable to perform a handstand or regular push-up and you're not likely to be able to do the 90-degree push-up.

The first step is to be able to perform an ordinary push up, then handstand , and finally a handstand push-up. After that, you might be capable of mastering the 90 degree push-up.

There are many advantages of bodyweight progress. This includes avoiding injuries and strengthening your body and overall physique, improving control over your movements, and developing the general knowledge of how to progress to more challenging exercises.

Going directly to an exercise isn't possible, it could result in injury to yourself. It is possible to be able to pull a muscle or fracture bones. It is essential to understand the proper way to operate any equipment and what type of form to choose and the amount your body can take.

A slower pace could also bring about faster progression. This is due to the fact that when you are working various muscles in different ways, the entire body will be working as opposed to the specific area of your body that's being engaged when you attempt to complete that more difficult movement repeatedly.

You should also consider that you can gain more control and control in your actions faster and also. If you work all over your body and carefully, you'll become more proficient and agile. It is because of a simple concept that we've been slogging around for long periods of duration "Practice is the best way to perfect." If you practice more you perform a single movement and the more proficient you master it. The more you do yoga-like movements, the more stable your flexibility, balance, and coordination will become.

Moving in different ways also helps you to learn more about the way your body moves. It also gives you a variety of exercises. Repeating the same move repeatedly can cause you to be bored. If your workout leaves you feel bored, then you're not going to be motivated to exercise for long! That means the goals you have set for yourself won't be worth the effort.

Chapter 7: Push-Ups

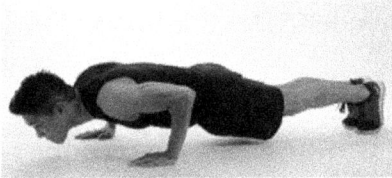

Push-ups are among the most used exercises for bodyweight currently. It doesn't take an expert on health and fitness to understand the meaning of a push-up. It's likely that you've performed a few.

The basic, standard push-up requires you to keep your weight on your toes and hands, and raise yourself, and then lower yourself again, without letting your body sink towards the ground. This workout builds strength in your upper body as well as the torso. It also strengthens your shoulders, wrists, tightens the core and improves your capacity to create muscles that are tight throughout your body.

The whole chapter will be devoted to the push-up. It will also cover more challenging variations which you'll perform once you've learned the fundamentals.

The Standard Push-up

There are numerous variations on the push-up you shouldn't be able to confidently begin working with them without having mastered the basic version. It's important to begin by perfecting the standard push-up before you attempt the more advanced ones.

Step 1: Balance your body with your toes and hands. Hands should sit shoulder-width apart, and the rest of your body should be in an erect line.

Step 2: As you face towards the forward direction and your eyes pointing towards the future take a few seconds to lower your elbows, and bend them to bring your body down to the ground. Your chest should be as close to the ground as it are able to manage. Your elbows can be allowed to disengage from your body.

Step 3: Take a break for a second , then push your chest upwards to make sure your arms straight once more.

Perform as many as three sets of 10, but in case you're not strong enough to do this, you should do 5-10 reps. Be sure to work an extra little bit each day to build up your strength.

*Note:

If you're not strong enough to push-up, you could begin by using a raised platform to push off from instead of lying flat on the floor. This helps you push against gravity much easier. You can also begin by placing your knees on the floor. This will help reduce the burden you must carry, while also gradually strengthening your upper body.

Variations of Push-ups

Like we said the calisthenics exercise relies on your body weight as a resistance. Therefore, you need to increase the level of difficulty as you progress. It is essential to make it more difficult the muscles are able to perform the effort. This is why you'll see that calisthenics comes with a myriad of variations of a single exercise that can be difficult to perform.

Here are some variations of push-ups.

Large and Close Grip

If you notice that you are getting stronger when you do your standard push-ups, and you can do three 10 sets, the most straightforward alternatives you can go to are the close and wide grip push-ups. By altering the posture on your hands, you're also modifying the muscles that are active.

The wide grip can make the chest muscles work harder The close grip strengthens the arm muscles and triceps.

The Wide-Grip Stairs are:

1: Place your hands in the normal beginning position to perform the push-up however, this time you should have your hands as far apart as you can.

2. Bend your elbows, and then bring your chest back, while maintaining all your other body parts as straight as you can.

3: Lower your body down as far as you possibly can (try to allow your chest to be in contact with the ground) before lifting your chest up.

Begin by working toward doing three sets of 10 repetitions.

Steps to close grip:

1: Once more, you'll need to take the normal push-up position, however the hands must be in close proximity. The tips of the fingers and your thumbs should be fingers should be touching when you place your hands down on the ground. They should be perpendicular to your center chest.

2. Again Bend your elbows and lower your chest while maintaining the body in a straight line.

3. Keep going downwards as far as you are able or until your chest is on the floor.

Continue to push upwards until you're back at the starting position.

Begin by working up to three sets of 10.

Fingertip Push-up and Wrist Pull-up

The fingertip push-up is an alternative of push-ups that specifically concentrates on the hands and fingers. This variant strengthens and strengthens your fingertips and hands that are essential to the progression of calisthenics. It is essential to have strong hands when you plan on performing certain of the more challenging exercises.

A wrist press-up similar to the fingertip version, increases the strength of the wrists, which is which is a joint that is relatively weak in the body.

Fingertip Push-up

Step 1: Sit in the standard push-up position however, instead of using the palms of your hands, place the weight of your body on your fingers. Spread your fingers. Because the thumb joint is stronger than the different fingers let your thumb carry the majority of the weight.

Step 2: Lower yourself down to the ground by bent elbows. Make sure you maintain the remaining part of your body tight and straight.

Step 3: After you've brought your chest to the lowest level you can or let it be in contact with the floor, push it upwards.

Try to complete at minimum 10 repetitions.

*Note: To improve difficulty in this particular variatlon, you should try using less and fewer fingers as you advance.

Push-ups for the wrist

Step 1: Starting from the traditional starting point of a standard push-up, lie your knees down on the ground instead of your hands, hold your body by using the fingers' backs. Your hands should be pointed toward the.

Step 2: Trying to keep your hands as straight as it can be bend your elbows and try to bring your chest close to the ground. Making sure your hands are as flat as they can make sure that you're as steady and comfortable as is possible.

Step 3: Once you have formed this position, and push your chest upwards until your arms are straight as possible.

Take note of being cautious when performing this exercise as your wrist can be a weak point for a large number of people. This exercise should be done with care.

Wall Push-up

This variation of the push-up increases resistance in the back as well as the difficulty overall of the workout. As you are aware, lifting the position of your upper body during push-ups can make it simpler. In addition, elevating the position of your lower back makes it even more difficult.

The wall push-up could appear easy enough since you're pushing up with your feet set against the wall. It can be quite difficult but the force on your shoulder that you use to push your feet up against the wall needs to be sufficient to keep you going.

Step 1. When you are facing the wall, you'll need to get into the normal push-up position with your feet in front of the wall. Lock your arms, and gradually walk your feet to the wall until they're in line to your shoulder. This is your starting point.

Step 2. Bend your elbows, then lower your chest until you are on the floor. While doing this, take your steps slowly down. Make sure that you remain as straight while doing this.

Step 3: After you've lower your chest to the ground, push it back up. Your feet should climb up the wall in tiny steps until you return to your original position.

Do at five reps at.

Note: The difficulty of this task means that you may encounter certain issues.

First, you might notice that your back is falling down, and an arch develops within your lower back. This indicates that your core muscles aren't yet robust enough, but it can be strengthened with time. If you feel that you're not capable of doing any reps , you can start from the beginning position and hold it for the length of time you are able to.

In the second, you may notice your feet moving away off the wall. This indicates that there's not enough pressure to hold your feet firmly to the floor. You'll need push back a little more to keep your foot upright.

If you'd like to increase the difficulty of this exercise, you can simply place your hands nearer to the wall. This makes exerting effort harder.

Chapter 8: What is Calisthenics?

Basic Questions answered

In this chapter, the very first in the text, we'll explore the fundamentals of calisthenics to help you grasp the subject. Calisthenics is one the most ancient forms of exercise. Exercise equipment and gyms are the latest inventions, and were not in use until a few years before. People would put in more effort to lose weight engaging in vigorous exercise and didn't rely on specific equipment or machinery.

The current scenario is completely different. From models to bodybuilders everyone loves making use of tools, like barbells and dumbbells, to shed weight. It's rare for individuals to begin calisthenics since they believe that using equipment will yield greater results more quickly. But, calisthenics is the basis for shaping the body and creating the body's core.

The only place that calisthenics remains a prominent part of the fitness routine is the military. Military personnel from a country tend to use calisthenics in order to strengthen their bodies to prepare to take on the most difficult physical challenges that may be faced. Calisthenics will help them improve their mental and physical strength thus enabling to tackle any obstacle or challenge that comes their way. These soldiers don't think about their appearance, and concentrate on building their strength to combat in the combat. But, as many can see, a good physique is a result of this type of training. Similar to regular individuals who do calisthenics will can increase their stamina, strength and physical endurance and also reduce total body fat.

If you're overweight and struggling to lose weight, the best way to beat it is engaging in a rigorous calisthenics workout. The regimen can be planned to suit your needs and be flexible to stay on track. Be assured that you'll be able to complete it if in a position to not have time to workout, because you can make do with the time required to complete calisthenics workouts to achieve the desired outcomes. By committing to it for 15 minutes per day you'll see substantial and lasting effects. You'll only need free space and loose clothes to start the exercises. No special equipment or clothes are required, but perhaps access to a nearby park with pull-up bars, or perhaps a gym station. The best part is that it's cost-free!

Here are some guidelines to follow in order to make callsthenics efficient.

Be constant

The most important thing is to ensure that you are consistently following the program for the greatest outcomes. According to health experts It is best for people to select exercises that can be done at least 4 or 5 times per week, as opposed to an exercise that is strenuous and may abandon within three days. If you choose exercises they can only do once per week typically will injure themselves when their bodies undergo an intense workout that could result in tears and wear.

Plan systematized

Create a plan that is systematic and stick to it until it's easier for you body adapt to your exercise routine. If you begin by too much, it could become challenging for the body to adjust to the routine. Many times, they abandon the exercise due to the extreme nature of it. Start by beginning with easy and moderate exercises that are simple to follow. Gradually increase the intensity the workout and select those which are appropriate for your body. Be sure to use this as your own motivation and stay on top of your exercise program. Keep in mind that it's important to limit the number of reps to more than 10 times per week, since it could be extremely strenuous for your body. Ask a health expert or a gym instructor to assist to plan your exercise program in case you have medical issues or have any other issues.

Take a good night's sleep.

A good amount of rest between exercise sessions is crucial. This allows your body to recuperate from your exercise routine and may lead to lower stress. Many people do not realize that their bodies begin to slim down in the recovery phase after working out, but not immediately after the workout. It is therefore essential to rest between workouts to ensure it becomes easier to shape your body. If you treat your workout like a continuous engine, your body will be challenging to recover, and gain endurance and strength.

Ideally, it is recommended to take a break for 30 seconds between workout sets. Utilize a timer or timer to record time , making it easier to break up the workouts. Give yourself a break of two days between two exercises. This can be used to engage in less strenuous activities like yoga and Pilates. However, you must not do any intense poses because the purpose is to allow your body enough time to heal from the previous day's working out. Be conscious of the body's limits and follow it because otherwise, you could be hurting yourself.

Be alert at signs that indicate fatigue because it's a sign of working too hard, or overtraining. If you experience any of these symptoms and you are experiencing fatigue, it is recommended to quit the workout or reduce the intensity of your routine. Continued practice of the same routine could adversely affect your health advancement or more seriously, you may decide to stop doing the routine altogether and lose any value from getting started from the beginning.

Breathing properly

The most crucial aspects of exercising is to pay attention to the quality of your breathing. It is crucial to breathe in a controlled manner to get the maximum effort possible during the workout routine. The oxygen that you inhale increases the energy levels of your body and also improves the coordination of your muscles. In general it is necessary to breathe in while contracting your muscles , and then exhale as you expand the muscles.

Intensity is the key

The majority of people who engage in calisthenics workouts believe that the amount of repetitions is more important in comparison to the intensity exercises. However, this isn't the case since it's the intensity that is important. Five repetitions of vigorous exercise is more effective than ten reps of exercises with low intensity. It is therefore essential to concentrate on the strength of the exercise opposed to the quantity. Keep in mind that all exercises must be done properly in order to prevent injury as well as encourage maximum fitness.

Keep it fascinating

One of the main tips that fitness enthusiasts can offer to stay consistent exercising with calisthenics is to keep it as exciting as is possible in order to overcome monotony. A lot of people take the exercises with great enthusiasm however, they end up dropping halfway through because they find it difficult or boring. To avoid this it is recommended to choose workout routines which are filled with energy and change them every now and then to keep your interest up. You could make a schedule of exercises you do for a week and then switch it up the following week. It is believed that the body could at times begin to adapt to certain exercises, rendering them useless. Therefore, it is recommended to mix up your exercises to avoid this from occurring.

Improve mental stamina

One of the main benefits of calisthenics training is that it aids in enhancing mental power. This is why it is that a lot of military personnel from different countries use this kind of training to build their troops' mental strength as well as prepare for the most difficult obstacles. It is necessary to have this type of training to keep up with your exercises till you have reached the goal you want to reach. If you can keep it up during the initial two months, it's more easy to keep going. When you are comfortable with the routine, you will be able to test your body's limits for the sake of testing your strength.

Make sure you eat right

It's a given that it is vital to consume a balanced diet while exercising to build a healthy and strong body. A lot of people exercise regularly without eating a proper diet and suffer due to this inattention.

If you eat right and exercise regularly, you are able to build a strong and healthy body which can perform the proper exercises and build stronger muscles that will effectively reduce the amount of fat within your body. Your hard work is wasted when you don't take your food in a healthy way. Your body's immune system will begin to weaken and your digestive system will be affected.

If you are going to do calisthenics, you need to eat a diet that is high in nutrients, such as carbohydrates as well as fats and proteins. They'll supply your body proper amount of nutrients needed to build your body up and give it the energy to perform the calisthenics exercise routine.

One of the most important nutrients to include into the diet of your choice is protein. Protein is essential for healthy growth of muscles and can supply an individual with growth to change your physique. However, this shouldn't mean that you should only focus on protein and neglect other nutrients. There must be some balance between them in order to give your body with the appropriate level of strength and endurance to perform calisthenics exercise. If you just increased your daily protein intake to 0.8grams per pounds of body weight, I am sure you'll notice an enormous change in your the body's composition within as short as one week.

If you're planning to follow a specific diet, like the ketogenic diet, it will be essential to select the appropriate type of food. It is possible to speak with an expert in nutrition to devise the right meal plan appropriate for your body's requirements.

Water must be given a lot of importance in eating a balanced diet. Drink as much water as you can to make it easy for your body to dissolve and flush out the toxins and nutrients out of your body. Eat fresh foods as well as drink lots of fluids to ensure optimal performance.

In the same way it's obvious and ideal to stay away from excessive nicotine and caffeine, because they could negatively affect your health and hinder your exercise routine. In this regard having a moderate dose of caffeine can be beneficial. Caffeine serves as the base of the majority of pre-workout supplements and fat burners. These provide users that extra boost during their workout and increase metabolism. If you drink too much, you may get stomach ulcers, heart palpitations and lose focus, which , as you'll observe, hinders the effects we desire.

Chapter 9: Train Like A Calisthenics King:

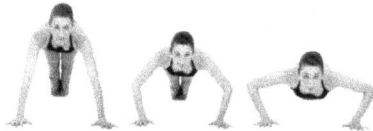

Stretching:

Many people are unaware of that stretching can be beneficial, or the need for an exercise pre- and post stretching routine. Stretching can prevent injuries, it's widely known and the term is used in every gym and for the right reasons. Stretching can boost your metabolism and triggers the basic muscle contraction mechanisms specifically of the muscles engaged in the intense workout routine that follows. It is also a good way to strengthen your cardiovascular system in order to gradually increase in the workload of your heart.

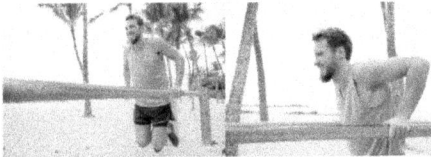

Stretching improves flexibility. You notice that you get up and your instinctual reaction would be stretching? It's your body's way of encouraging and prepare for moving. Stretching prior to and after exercise helps keep your muscles flexible A lot of people aren't keen to stretch due to it being generally associated with a dull throbbing sensation especially if you've already increased your size. However, the good thing is that you will become accustomed to it and eventually feeling the rush of chemicals after exercise and the sensation of tension dissolving away from the body.

There isn't a set rule for how to stretch or the length you must stretch, but the post-workout stretch is recommended for bodyweight lifters since there is less chance of injury during this type of exercise. Also, any pain that occurs after exercise is typically a result of an ingredient called lactic acid, which builds up as a result of exercising. Thus, stretching following a workout reduces the amount of this chemical and relieves the pain.

Muscle groups that you must be working:

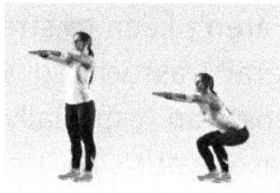

Arm muscles:

The muscles of the rotator cuff such as biceps, deltoids, and brachialis are the primary muscles that must be activated. Simple wrist and arm rotations suffice for this.

The back muscles:

Trapezius as well as latisamus dorsi the rhomboids. These muscles can be stretched out by taking your arms from your body and raising them over your head in a manner similar to birds spreading their wings before striking the ballerina pose. Repeating this move many times.

The abdominal muscles:

Obliques and recti. These muscles can be worked by securing your fingers with your chest facing forward and letting your elbows extend to towards the side. Then, shift your shoulders in a rotational direction by pushing your left elbow forwards and then an upward motion of your left elbow. Repeat this a few times. This is a fantastic exercise that will strengthen your core muscles. You can actually feel the heat within a short time.

leg muscles:

The primary leg muscles you must stretch are the quads, hamstrings and calves. They are all used to perform simple lunges.

The simplest, most efficient and, by far, the most effective stretch routines typically involve traditional jumping jacks, often referred to by the name of star jumps. The jumping jacks are a great exercise for all muscle groups , and increase your heart rate . This makes for the ideal pre- and post-workout exercise routine.

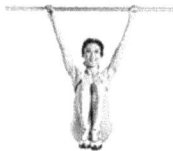

The essentials:

This section will focus on the various exercises used in Calisthenics and, while many of them are things that you've heard of, it's the proper form and the way they work out that makes Calisthenics an amazing exercise. While they are not as complicated as they appear, these exercises form the base for the incredible martial arts moves utilized by masters like Bruce Lee. If done correctly you'll see the reasons these exercises are employed as a basic tool for training any other sport exercises.

Calisthenics are a type of fundamental exercises. They progress to higher levels by changing on the exercises. The exercises are:

pull-ups: Pull-ups require a pull-up bar as which is mentioned in the equipments. You utilize your upper body strength and a strong core to push your body up while flexing your arms. This will strengthen your muscles, arms, and back.

Push-ups: Get down on all fourswith your with your arms shoulder-width apart. elevate your knees off of the ground based on your fitness level and keep your stomach off the floor, and hold your position as if you were in a straight "plank" (hence"planking"). name "planking" it is an excellent exercise that builds the arms and core) Bend your elbows and lower yourself to the ground after the same process by stretching the elbows and using your core muscles to maintain your posture while you lift your body off of the floor.

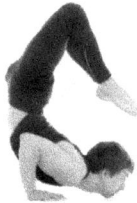

Be sure to do it slow. A typical push up should not take more than one second

Dips: This exercise utilizes the dip bar and can help to strengthen your triceps muscles. Hold both sides of your dip bar and push your arms to stretch to the elbow joint so that you can lifting your weight off the ground, then lower yourself by extensing your arms.

Inverted rows: place your dip bar at your waist then grab a grip that is wide enough for your shoulders and begin being suspended from the bar. You can move your elbows to place your chest in close proximity to the bar, then raise your elbows until you return to your starting the position.

Squats: Begin in a standing posture with your feet spread wide and then contract your core muscles by bend your knees to the point that you were planning to sit, and then returning to the starting position.

hanging knee raises: Using your pull-up bar, begin by hanging straight from it , then, tighten your core and raise your knees towards your abdomen, lifting them off the ground . After that return to the starting in the same position.

You can do variations of this exercise by moving your legs to the left or right side to strengthen your muscles in the obliques.

Many people do this exercise with their legs in a position known as raising their legs with a hanging device.

Hand stands-Variation:

You may begin to introduce modifications when you realize that your training routine isn't producing a sweat, and you are performing them like you would an easy stretch routine. at this point you should be seeing improvements in the strength of your body as well as overall body weight. These are the most commonly used variants of the fundamentals:

It may appear hard, but after working it out and beginning with the help from the wall, you could be amazed by the various options you'll be able to achieve by placing your feet on the ground and your legs suspended in the air.

one-arm push-ups are an intermediate-level pushup that you can attempt once you've learned the basics of the push-up. You can perform the basic push-up by alternate arms. This means that only one arm is able to support the entire body weight.

Other push ups include:

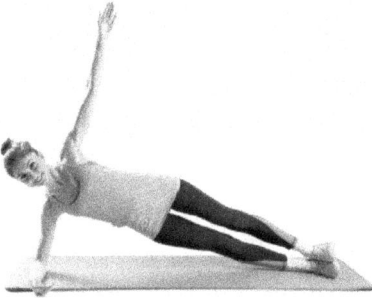

prop your legs up on higher ground in order to put more weight on your arms and trunk This can be followed by pushups with one arm propped up

Wide grip push-ups: in which your arms are further apart than your shoulder width when doing an exercise, this is the most challenging method of doing the pushup.

One-arm pull-ups is a tougher type of pull-ups in which you only use one arm to support your body weight completely.

jumping squats, also known as jumping squats are a method of incorporating aerobics into Calisthenics weight training, but coming back to the beginning of a squat following a the sitting position, by jumping and extensing your knees. This is a great exercise for glutes and is also incorporated into the cross-fit "burpee" exercise.

Oblique handing knee raises A form of knee raises hanging from the ceiling that instead of lifting your knees straight toward your abdomen, you concentrate in pulling them toward the opposite part of the body, while the knees are curved towards your abdomen, and then alternate sides.

Plank variant:

sideplank: place yourself on the side while you plank so that your whole weight is supported by just the facet of your body, while you're facing in the opposite direction. Then, lift your free arm into the air to balance yourself.

Leg lift plank: Plank while lifting alternative legs off the ground.

Arm lift plank: Planking while lifting one arm off of the ground.

Plank downhill: supporting your legs on a surface that is elevated.

Wall March plank: Use a the push-up bar to grip when you lift your legs off the floor and then push your heels up against the wall while you plank.

One knee squat is a basic squat that requires one knee being stretched while the other knee is extended to squat. This is referred to as the single knee squat.

Advanced:

Once you've learned the basic levels of bodyweight training, it's time to progress towards the techniques of the elite. These movements require the use of the basic Calisthenics movements and keeping the correct shape for a specified amount of duration (recall the long isometric contraction that we talked about in earlier chapters) These exercises will can really get you into the top ranks and will help you compete with weightlifters. These exercises are an exercise in coordination and balance. They also integrate the lessons you've learned during your training.

Dragon flag:

The name was coined by the creator of the movement, Bruce Lee, Dragon Flag is a well-known Calisthenics move that is incredibly effective on your body's center. It was also featured as a scene in Rocky IV movie, and after you've performed it, you'll understand the reason!

You've now gained enough strength from your variations to master this maneuver. The time it takes to hold the position will improve with time, so don't stress you're on the way to becoming the best!

Begin by lying down on a bench. Get in a position that is ready by putting your hands against the bench at least the height of your head, and then gradually straight back and take your hips, legs and abdominals off the bench by stepping upwards on your shoulders. Slowly lower yourself until you're not in contact with the bench, and then hold that the position until you return to your starting position.

Pistol is used to squats

A more advanced version of squatting in which you begin with the normal starting position of the single knee squat and then while in the that squatting position, reduce yourself to the point that your bent knee is fully flexed, while your other knee is fully extended, while being taken off from the ground. Maintain the in this position.

This is a more difficult variation of pistol squats. The athlete uses a kettle-bell to stand. Make sure you be able to complete it without the kettle-bell first, then you can try it with a kettle-bell to increase your strength

Handstand push ups with hand-held devices

Beginning in the normal handstand position, lower your head down to the ground by bending your elbows. Then return to the normal handstand position by extending your elbows.

Start by with the wall. Once you are able to complete them correctly and be competent enough to complete more than 20 times, you could try this without the wall . This exercise can help you increase your balance, and also..

PLANCHE:

The most advanced version of the plank, where you maintain your position in a plank with your hips, abdomen and knees elevated off the floor. Begin by getting into a the normal plank position, then pull your knees to the side so that they rest on the crooks of your elbows. you utilize your abdominals and arms to support the weight (this is known as the frog posture) From here, you extend your knees so that your hips are raised off the ground and you're a straight plank that you can balance with your arms. Keep your position.

Tips for beginners:

In the process of preparing for a pull up Start by using an stool or a chair to sit on during an exercise called a pull up. This reduces the distance you need to go to the top by making the exercise more easy.

Start working towards a push-up with pushups against walls, and then lower yourself to chairs or counters which are higher than the ground until you are able to build enough strength that you can perform pushups off the ground.

Planking: Begin by doing 20 second planks. Then work your way to a 3-2 minute planks, adding an increment of 20 seconds every day.

A regular increase in intervals can help you build more strength.

Make sure that your back is straight, and remember to breathe.

Examples of Routines:

Although you are able to create your own routines using the fundamental, variant and advanced exercises , it's beneficial to have a reference in order to know how to go from the basic to the advanced level of training. It is possible to do this through interval training that involves quick repetition of basic movements or perform slow and sustained, basic moves to build up strength to perform the more advanced movements. Examples:

Beginning routine-intervals:

Pull-ups for 1 minute. Perform as many pull-ups you can. Followed by 15 seconds of relaxation

Inverted rows 1 minute of inverted rows, then fifteen seconds rest

Dips: 1 minute of the maximum amount of dips you can do followed by 15 seconds of intervals

Push-ups: Maximum number of dips that you can complete in a minute followed by 15 minutes of rest.

Squats: The most number of quick-paced squats within 1 minute, followed by three minutes of rest before you begin the whole routine.

Repeat the entire process as many amount of times within a half hour or whatever time you feel at ease starting with.

Beginning routine- classic reps:

Circuit A:

Pull-ups 30 times.

Dips 30 times

Squats 30 times

Circuit B:

Inverted rows: 20 times

Push-ups 20 times

Hanging knee rises: 20 times

One arm plank 20 times

Crunches: 20 times.

Do two circuits, each with a break of 1 minute between circuits.

In order to train for advanced or intermediate levels, you can utilize the variations and advanced techniques in your routine of basic training after you've mastered these.

Chapter 10: Bodyweight Specifics

When you begin your journey to lose weight, you must to decide what your objectives are. If you don't set goals, you'll have no motivation to pursue anything. The goals you set are likely to be centered around the following:

What do you'd like to accomplish?

Are you looking to become stronger, bigger or maybe a bit of both?

What are you hoping to excel at?

Setting your goals ought to be easy and straightforward since generally people seek strength, endurance or size, specific skills or a mix of these. It is worth noting that strength is beneficial to all the things you're trying to get better at, so when you're a mix of these, it's important to focus on your strengths first.

After you've identified your goals, your next task is to select the exercises that will help you achieve the capabilities you would like to develop. Because of the numerous exercise routines that are included in bodyweight fitness, there is no way that you'll be able do all of them, even though there is an abundance of transferrable goals which are similar. It is suggested to pick at least five goals which you can start working towards.

The way bodyweight exercises work

Fitness with bodyweight does not consist of endless presses or rounds of simple exercises. Training with bodyweights is a real resistance training.

Strength

To increase your strength it is recommended to do 3 to 5 sets that includes 3-8 repetitions of heavy exercises, with will give you as much rest as you'd like between sets. Your goal is to build up the resistance level between your exercises.

Muscle Size

For a larger muscle mass, you must complete three sets, 8 to 12 repetitions of intense exercises, with a rest of two mins between sets.

Endurance

For endurance , you need to do the workout you'd like to get better at and perform lots of them!

The ranges of repetitions listed are pretty random, and this is all up to personal preference and there's a lot of overlap. Three sets of 3-8 repetitions will help build muscle, whereas three sets that have 8 to 12 repetitions also covers the strength. Beginners should start with three sets and 5-8 repetitions.

The most important thing is to master the art of increasing the strength of an exercise, and this is accomplished by using patterns. It is defined as a sequence of exercises that are the same type/.group in which each exercise is somewhat more challenging than the previous. The first exercise is to work through the exercise you are working on until you've gained enough strength to perform the first workout and then the next exercise for a few times. Continue working on exercise 2 till you're ready to begin working for the final exercise.

This is a fantastic concrete example:

If you've chosen to do the pushup option but you can't perform a pushup, begin with a pushup on walls (vertical pushup) after you've mastered this , move onto pushups that are on a surface with a raised edge like the desk (incline pushups) and once you're confident in this, you are able to begin regular pushups.

The sequence of events in this case is:

Vertical pushups, the incline pushup Regular pushups.

Be prepared , as you'll discover that you are unable to increase your the difficulty of each workout because the progression steps are too challenging. If you want to increase your difficulty , you may also increase repetitions. In the majority of cases, you'll be able to move up when you have completed 3x10 of the exercise you are currently doing.

Training with bodyweight

Muscle development through bodyweight training

You can build muscle using the bodyweight exercise and this is the point where diet plays a role. Diet is the 80% factor in the way you look , and to build muscle (provided you're at your weight of your recommended) you'll need to take in more food. The training to build muscles will require you to follow a the same progressions that you perform for three sets, with between 8 and 12 repetitions for each exercise, and then resting for no more than one and a quarter minutes between sets.

Work on strength and skill

Skill work is things that require lots of practice to allow you to gain proficiency. Skill work is not a job that has any strength as the primary component.

Handstands are a great illustration of the skill. You need strength to be able to do it, but balance is an important factor. Beginning users do not have the strength required to stand up. They will be mainly working on their handstand's strength and balance is not an important role, therefore for the beginner, a handstand will be a form of strength training. As the beginner gains strength, the handstand becomes more about balance since the strength of the hand is not an essential factor, and this is the time when the beginner's handstand turns into an exercise in skill.

It is recommended to separate the work of strength and skill. The skill work you do is supposed to be simple and not tiring to ensure that you can get maximum benefit from your time working on. The skills you are practicing should be done prior to the strength workout and are the basis of your warm-up This means that you won't get tired during your work out. Make use of a set number of repetitions or a set duration of time to master.

Every exercise that requires greater strength than anything else is not considered skill work. This means that moves like handstands or L-sits are categorized as strengthening, but that will only be the case initially. It is crucial to dedicate time to training things like handstands constitute a part of the final objective.

Equipment

There will be a need for equipment to do pull-ups because they are essential for correcting imbalances that a majority of people suffer from. This type of apparatus can be a branch of a tree or stairwell. It can also be used with towels, ropes and so on. They can be thrown over anything that is strong if impossible to hold onto the tree branch, etc.

In the event of completing rows inverted, hanging them from a sturdy table, tree , etc. can be used to make equipment. Alternately, you can utilize a broom, or any other straight object that is strong and placed between two chairs.

To dip, you can use the backs of two chairs. Just remember to place things that are heavy on the chairs in case you believe they could slide over when you're working with them.

The ideal place to practice L-sits is the floor.

You can also make yourself equipment, if are an artist. The only thing you need to be aware of is that it's secure.

Progress

There are numerous websites that are free and you can find out more about the different types of progressions that are found in various exercises.

Leg work

There aren't a lot of leg exercises to do when it comes to training with body weight. Squats or leg curl variations will be all you need to choose from, however these are good enough and provide advantages for those looking to improve their leg muscles.

Additional leg exercises can be found by using barbells for training. Calf raises are not included because they aren't difficult, and they do not provide any progress without adding weight.

We will therefore focus on the many ways you can incorporate squats as well as deadlifts in your bodyweight workout. Two of the best alternatives:

Include squats into your workouts and add deadlifts at least once per week at the conclusion of your training.

Squats are can be incorporated into one of the workouts, and deadlifts as part of the third workout to complement your leg exercises.

The suggested exercise for squats is three sets of 5 repetitions , and for deadlifts, 1 set of five repetitions. It is suggested to complete 1 to 3 sets of squats and deadlifts with the use of a lighter weight to warming up before continuing by doing squats and deadlifts.

Development

When your progress slows down or you reach a plateau in your beginning routine, it's the right time to shift to an intermediate regimen. The first changes will be focused on the frequency of your week and you'll be performing specific exercises, giving you more time to recover while making the transition to the concept of deloading.

To implement this you must:

1.) Select a set of exercises and a repetition target

It is dependent on your goals for strength and endurance, muscle size, or strength and also different amounts of repetitions. The recommended amount for beginners is still 5-8 repetitions, while the 3 to 5 repetitions are perfect for more challenging exercises, with the set remaining similar in the range 3 to 5.

2.) Choose a template from the below templates or one that you've done your own research on

Full body, two days two workouts that combine 1 push, 1 pulling exercise and 1 leg exercise and 1 the core exercise.

Split push/pull - Two exercises that both include 3 or more push exercises, and one leg exercise. The second will include 3 or more pull exercises and 1 leg extension.

3 workouts that include 3 push exercises as well as hold support work. The final workout consists of two to three exercises for the legs and core work.

Volume/light/heavy - 3 workouts that include a variety of repetitions, progressions and repetitions. Each workout consists of one push, one pull, 1 leg, and 1 x fundamental exercises. This volume exercise is performed with more repetitions, which typically fall within the 10-12 range. This light exercise is completed by using a more gradual progression with moderate repetitions usually in the 5-8 range. The more intense workout is performed by using the most effective progressions with fewer repetitions, typically within the range of 3 to 5.

3.) Pick your time for your workout

Your workout routine must be part of your routine, and the following are two ways to do this:

A week of 3 days with an off day in between. This is the standard Monday/Wednesday/Friday layout and you alternate through each workout

2 days on, 1 day off. This is the arrangement that allows you to perform two exercises in succession and then the rest day. This is the most effective timing schedule for the split templates mentioned in the second paragraph above, since it is more compact between days.

4.) Select specific exercises that will fill in your template

It is recommended to check your performance in a specific exercise before it can incorporate into your routine. Start by warming up and then test your movements on every progression you intend to utilize. It is important to select the exercise that you're capable of finishing the number of repetitions that is appropriate basis to have good technique. If you discover you're not able to finish the required repetitions, you need to choose a more gradual progression or vice versa, if you can handle more repetitions.

5) Organize your exercises

Start with the exercise you are most eager to improve. Do 3 to five sets of this exercise and then rest for whatever time is necessary prior to moving to the next step of your workouts. Remember that whether you've used both pulls and pushes that these must be rotated.

6) Make sure you have the skill before the strength

Skill work is specific to sport and assists you in reaching your goals. Skill work requires no or low fatigue, but is more difficult to complete in the time. Any task that requires more practice and requires effort is considered skilled work. The most common recommendation for considering skills work is to do the exercises for a certain period of time that includes your time to rest. Concentrate on resting and making every attempt successful that are not too tiring.

The handstands as well as L sits are fundamental skills that have advantages that are to work on. The ability to balance and move with agility is great additions to any intermediate stage. Activities like yoga trees, simple leg lifts of the calf, etc. can help build these skills.

Do not forget anything that demands more strength than any other task is not considered as the work of a skilled worker.

7.) Warm up

The goal of a warming up is to heat your entire body to enable you to exercise using all moves while engaging muscles in a way that they're rarely utilized. If you're experiencing mobility issues that prevent you from engaging in the exercises now is the perfect time to address them. Begin your warm-up with exercises that bring your blood flow.

8) Conditioning

While it is not mandatory Conditioning is recommended and can include exercises like cycling, running or jumping rope. Conditioning can be done during times when you're not training for strength or added towards the final part of your training.

9) It's time to go

Have fun as you begin your training!

The routines consist of warming up and skill work, as well as exercises for strength as well as a few workouts and stretching can consume many hours and many people don't have the time.

The best method to cut down on time is to do your mobility and flexibility on days off. These activities are not demanding and can even aid your recovery.

The second is strengthening work. If you're already performing mobility exercises on days off and your strength routine takes too long you may want to think about joining your workouts. If, for instance, you do pushups and rows with a 3-minute break between sets, these can be combined by doing one set of pushups after which you rest for 1.5 minutes, and then completing the same set of rows, before taking a 1.5 minutes to rest. This is because the pairing does not require a lot of muscles that are overlapping, so rowing won't have an enormous effect on what you're getting from pushups and the reverse is true.

If you're still feeling that you aren't getting enough time to complete your workout, think about removing some exercises or dividing the workload in different days for workouts.

Chapter 11: Diverse Kinds Of Calisthenic Exercises

Calisthenics are classified into 3 distinct types that will be discussed in the following section.

Lower Body Calisthenics, with specific examples:

The calisthenics type is focused on strengthening the lower parts of the body like knees, hips, limbs and ankles. Examples of calisthenics workouts that help build the lower part of your body are hover lunges, squatting, burpees.

Images of calisthenics for the lower part

Squat:

This kind of calisthenic is helpful to build up the thigh and knee.

Lunge:

This exercise is highly efficient for building muscles , such as calves, hamstrings, thighs, calves as well as glutes and hips.

Burpees:

This is an excellent workout to build muscle mass such as hips, thighs, back and knees. It can also go an extended way in building the chest and arm. Regularly doing burpees can have an impact on posture and bodybuilding.

II. Upper body calisthenics, and specific exercises:

This kind of calisthenics is focused on strengthening the upper region of your body, such as the chest, shoulder and back, arms, etc. Some examples of calisthenics for upper bodies include dips, pull-ups and push-ups and archers' pull-ups. handstand push-ups and skull crushers. benches dips and so on.

Images from upper-body Calisthenics

Push-ups:

This workout helps build and strengthen muscles in the upper portion of your body, such as your chest, back and shoulder muscles. It also strengthens abdominal muscles.

Pull-ups

This workout is designed to strengthen and build up your shoulders, back and arm (triceps and Biceps).

Dip:

This exercise is crucial for building abdominal muscles, chest and the triceps.

The essence:

This is a kind of calisthenics, which help strengthen and build the central region that is the core of our body. The center comprises of the pelvis, lower back and abdominal. Core exercises have a huge impact on building six packs. The most common core calisthenics exercises which will aid in building strong core muscles are legs lowers, planks dead-bug low backs, dragon flags, etc.

Below are photos of the most important exercises for calisthenics

Plank:

This workout is believed to be extremely beneficial to build and strengthen the lower pelvis, hips, and back (LHPC).

Dead Bug.

This workout is among the most effective methods to strengthen and build the abdominal muscles as well as your your core, which gives you an attractive and physical appearance. Dead bug requires you to lay flat on your back. After that, you turn your left knee to 90 degrees, with your right hand extended toward the upward direction. Reduce your right leg, left hand and the lower part of your body lightly and then bend your right hand and left knee upwards for the next step.

Lower back

Chapter 12: Calves & Shoulders

Calves

3 sets of 10-12 repetitions. 30-40 seconds rest between sets.

Execution: Stand with your feet approximately shoulder width apart. Your toes can be pointed in various directions while performing this exercise. In, out and back. This will allow you to build fully calve muscles from the inside out. Lift the sole of your feet, hold it for one count and squeeze towards the top. You could also do this exercise in a single leg.

Shoulders

3 sets, 10-12 repetitions per each exercise. 30-40 seconds rest between sets.

Front raises to help front dets

Execution: Hold one dumbbell each with your arms positioned over your body. Maintain your arms straight, but slightly bent when lifting arms up to shoulder level. Avoid swinging the arms. Lower the arms until they are at your their thighs, then repeat the move.

Side lateral raises for side delts.

Execution - Similar to front raises above , however the dumbbells are at your sides, not front of you.

Bent over laterals for rear delts.

Execution – Same as front and side raises with the exception that you'll be bent or seated. Arms should be raised until they reach the shoulder height.

Traps - 3 sets of 10-12 repetitions for each exercise. 30-40 seconds rest between sets.

Execution Shrugs. Relax your shoulders to the maximum extent you are able. As you hold your body steady by shrugging your shoulders slowly straight upwards to the highest point you can. Do not rotate your shoulders forward or backwards. Stop for a period of 3 to 3, and after that, slowly bring the dumbbells to their starting position. Concentrate on getting the weight up using the traps, not your Biceps.

It is not necessary to move the shoulders back or forward in shrugging exercises. The notion that this will help you isn't true. The best thing to do is shrug straight up as high as you can. Make sure to stop near the end of the exercise to reap the maximum benefits in the training. Be sure to not let your arms or body move upwards and downwards. The movements should be fluid and controlled throughout.

Chapter 13: Strategies for Fitness At Home and Getting Results

Be Consistent

Find out which timetable is most suitable for your needs. Keep it in your calendar and save it there.

. My preference is working out in the early hours of the day. However, on days when I workout from home, I go out in early in the morning to go to work. I prefer to schedule it with a show that I enjoy and follow my schedule. Don't be stressed when your life becomes an overwhelming burden. Get some family time in. Walks or lunges in the midst of a meticulous child, or do squats when cooking dinner or even doing a few laps up and down to the stairs in between meal prep.

Music

For some people who are struggling, the most difficult part of exercising from home can be the lack of motivation to work out. You must first create a domain on which you'll be using to use for your exercise. I have found that choosing a good Pandora station or creating an energetic playlist is the most effective among other methods for exercising at home. Music is a fantastic source of energy for exercising So make sure to turn it up and start the workout!

Set Goals

Make a plan for how you must meet. I recommend setting an alarm to remind you when you'd like to work out as an update to the week prior or something similar. You won't have to repeat it after the second week, but don't hesitate to utilize the strategy for the duration you require to stay in the right direction.

Get an expertly fitted

There are people on this world who have been educated in different steps that are rhythmic, running or walking They know how to position you in shoe that works most effectively for you. They will help you. The few hours you devote to learning towards the front will yield huge benefits, particularly if aren't injured and move around freely. (And we do refer to "afternoon"as your feet expand throughout the day, which is why you'd prefer not to get fitted at the morning in the morning.) The local multipurpose sporting goods store might not be the best place to need to go to for this. Look for a store that is able to supply their customers with the correct shoes. A reputable running shoe shop like this one will include treadmills, cameras and complete a full walk analysis for absolutely free. Make use of this service, and then make a purchase as much as you are able. They can't stay in operation if you make use of their diagnostic services. Then, go home and buy your shoes from the internet. Furthermore, if the small people who are aware of the dangers they're putting in, they'll quit their jobs, we all pay the price by being hurt more often. Another advantage of these local stores is that they usually let you return shoes after you have worn them, in the event that they don't match the way you expected This is an enormous help as you learn the intricacies of your footwear.

Have a few go-to workouts That you have memorized

Remember a small portion of your favorite schedules from magazines and websites for health. I've learned a few of my favorite exercises for strength by heart and I'm able to rely on them with no fail you find new workouts to add to the list. It's an all-encompassing and fantastic broad-based training program for your brain, too! I generally can perform my personal Yoga or Pilates practice whenever there's an hour or so to exercise my body. I also enjoy the set form of yoga known as Ashtanga which is a similar sequence of postures each time. If I'm not feeling motivation, I often practice the Ashtanga exercise so that I don't have to think about it too much. The standard Pilates Tangle exercise is an great option for me to try because I'm familiar with the pattern.

In particular, you should identify specifically your "why" and focus on your own the journey, not someone other's.

It's a huge element of remaining calm in a positive, steady, and predictable manner as you begin to exercise. Determine the reason why you are ready to integrate a regular fitness routine into your daily life and meet your goals Tanker. It might require some digging and must be meaningful enough for you to be able to rely on when you are tempted to stop. You might be able to remain conscious of your children and feel secure within your body, or just set aside the time to think about your health.

In the end, it should be about your goals and what is comfortable for you. If you're embarking on the path to fitness, it may be easy to get involved in what everyone else is doing. Remember that we all go at our own pace, and focus on what is best and most appealing to you and your body.

High-intensity exercise.

If you're beginning an exercises, it's recommended to start slowly such as, for instance, if you're cycling or running, build your endurance at least a month prior to starting any more intense exercise. This means that you should be working at a pace where you can talk easily without feeling exhausted. If you do have the foundation of determination then increase the intensity to increase the effectiveness of your exercise.

Make use of a fitness tracker

It's still a bit confusing however, I tend to do more and work out harder when I are wearing a fitness monitor. I love to organize challenges with my friends However I love to push myself to make progress as well. Most days that I exercise I can complete the 10k step. Some days, it may not happen.

Compound Exercises

Instead of working your muscles with exercises, like the curl of your bicep, extend the time you invest on a fitness routine by engaging in exercises that exercise multiple muscles simultaneously. By performing just a few exercises, you can achieve a full-body exercise. Another benefit is that your muscles are performing like they do in real life instead of working in isolation. A few amazing compound exercises include deadlifts, squats, good mornings, lunges and pushups and seat squeezes, lines, military presses, dips, pull-ups and much more.

Protein

A lot of people don't give thoughtful consideration to the protein they need for their muscles to rejuvenate. If you don't do this, you'll gain nothing from your exercise, since both cardiovascular and quality exercises require protein to build muscles. I suggest either whey protein shakes or natural foods.

Water

Be sure to drink plenty of water throughout the day. It takes time for your body's system to hold the water. Therefore, it isn't a good idea to drink before exercising. It is a good idea to drink water regularly throughout the entire day.

Carbs

Despite what the low-carb trend may claim that carbohydrates are our body's main source of energy. If you exercise regularly and require carbs or else you'll not have enough energy. If you do shakes, you should choose one that contains carbsand a banana is an amazing source of low-fiber/high-glycemic sugars you require to perform your training.

Shake Before Working Out

It's recommended to consume an energy drink with protein or carbs prior to your workout, and immediately following. The shake you drink prior to exercise boosts levels of amino acids into your muscles, thereby providing them with the squares of building they require. After your exercise, the shake will stimulate the development of muscles. Also, have a little carb/protein meal 60 minutes and a half following a workout . A food substitute bar could work well.

Dispose of the Distractions

Doggy, children, phones or whatever you can manage to keep things in check that could keep you busy before you start a exercise session at home.

Set a time when your spouse, friend or a neighbor will watch your children. Place your pets in a different room , and put your phones aside so that when you start your workout you'll be aware of your chance to finish it! There's nothing worse than getting distracted by social media or electronic gadgets.

Do not limit Your Area

If you're working out in your home does not mean that you must stay in your home. The exercise routine mentioned above is a good opportunity to take a trip outdoors, no matter if it's a course for running that you've planned out with an app such as RunKeeper or a quick bike ride in a nearby route. As reported by in the New York Times, there are many benefits to taking your workout outside whenever you are able to. There is no need to go outside for every workout however, make sure you mix it all in to keep your routine fresh.

Make it a public issue

Hold the telephone--literally, before you tweet, message, or gram your workout designs, read this: You will have a superior shot of actually working out if you remain quiet about them. A study suggests that social acknowledgement makes us less likely to delivering on our goals.

After you've completed your body, don't be afraid to shout it on social media. Take a photo of where you stand , or snap an emo-soaked selfie. If you talk about your progress and achievements, you'll gather a small group of team-promoters who can profit from that energized feeling whenever you're around training.

Chapter 14: Vital Practices that Will Ensure Success in Calisthenics

Focus

Concentration is an important factor in achieving your goals for exercise. It's much easier for your body improve when you are able to focus on the movements you perform while exercising. There are three kinds of concentration:

(i) Focus on the short-term(ii) Short-term focus - this is where you will learn to remain focused during your workout routine.

(ii) Midterm focus - This is when you regularly keep track of your routines for your workouts without missing a single day. This is achieved by doing this for several months.

(iii) Long-term focus - This when you adhere to your routines until you've attained your goals.

To help you focus better To improve your focus, you need to eliminate all distractions during your workout. Some examples of this are phones on your mobile and television. Also, you should avoid the new routines that are introduced each day and remain focused on what you are doing until the very end.

Consistency

Consistency is the ability to exercise regularly without slacking. In order for your body to grow you must remain focused on following the timetable for your workout. If you're planning to work out in the morning, start every day, without rethinking your plans.

Try your best to make it happen.

There is no easy way to live life. When you are doing anything you must make the effort to achieve the desired outcome. The same rules apply to your calisthenics exercises and you must be in an attitude of a goal-oriented person in order to master new skills faster and achieve your goal.

If you're finding it difficult to motivate yourself If you are struggling to motivate yourself, try purchasing calisthenics training video clips and allow the trainer to motivate you. Additionally, try picturing the body you would like and how awesome it would be to get it.

Controlling non-training-related factors

There are many other aspects in addition to your training that could affect the progress of your training, like your sleep habits and diet. So, it is important to have enough rest to allow your body time to rest and increase your energy levels. Also, make sure to adhere to good eating habits if you are looking to build up enough energy for different calisthenics workouts.

Patience

Nothing is ever done overnight. This is a well-known expression, but how many have the discipline to adhere to the rules to the letter? It's a very small number. Do not enter fitness with a quick fix mentality. It requires patience to reach your the goals you set. Keep in mind the nervous system requires time to adapt to the exercise you're doing, however, as time passes it will get stronger and can achieve the desired result.

Tip: Keep your eye on the prize will assist you to be patient . You can also create short-term goals that will help keep you focused.

Calisthenics Body Weight Training for Upper Body Usefulness

In this section, I'm going to guide you through various exercises that can help improve your upper body strength. In this instance, our primary areas of concern are your arms, abs and shoulders.

Abs

The abdominal muscles play an essential role in linking your body's upper part with your legs. They help keep your torso straight while walking or standing. The exercises I will teach you below will only require you to have sufficient space with a bench, pull-up bar, and an area to lie on. Now let's get straight into the exercises:

Dragon fly

Step 1: Sit down on the bench and place your eyes facing upwards.

Step 2: Extend your hands towards the top of your head and attach them to the bench to provide assistance.

Step 3. Engage your abdominal muscles to assist to lift your body. Remember that your body needs to be straight from your shoulders all the way to your knees.

Step 4. Once you're in the position you want to be, keep it for a few minutes, preferably for 20 seconds. the first time.

Step 5 Step 5: After 20 seconds then slowly lower your body, while keeping the straight line of your body.

6. Repeat this process 10 times.

Planks

Planks are a great exercise that will assist you in gaining an overall strength. Here's how you can accomplish it:

1. Lay flat on your back on the ground.

Step 2: Lift your back by supporting it by using your toes as well as your elbows as seen in the above picture.

Step 3: Stay at this point for twenty seconds, if you are just starting out. Repeat the entire exercise 15 times more each day.

If you're comfortable with the routine Try lifting one hand, one leg or both at the same time, while keeping that plank-like position.

Front lever

This is typically performed in the more advanced stages. This should be your long-term objective on the list of exercises you want to be completed.

Step 1: Locate an overhead bar and hang it onto it in the manner shown in the image above.

Step 2: Smooth your body until it is vertical to the ground.

Step 3: Keep this position until exhausted, then repeat the entire exercise 15 times more.

This exercise will strengthen your abs as well as your entire body.

Leg raise

Your abdominal muscles must be strong to raise your knees or your legs while doing this calisthenics workout. This workout will build the strength of your core.

Step 1: Locate an exercise bar that is pull-up and then hang it while you place your legs together and then stretch them outward.

Step 2. Flex the knees (knee raise) and then hold this position for 20 minutes. As you get stronger, you can try the leg raise. Instead of elevating your knees, lift your legs like the name implies.

Step 3: Repeat the exercise 10 times more for a total of two sets.

Other abdominal exercises include

The L-sit

Crunches

Leg pull-ins

V- sit ups

Flutter kicks

TIP: Consider establishing an exercise routine that you can organize it in the following way:

50 sit-ups, 5 minute leg holds 30 L-sit leg raises 50 hip side plank raises 25 reps of the dragon flag 75 leg raises, and 100 sit-ups.

Here's an image that shows the exercises can be used to strengthen your abs.

Arms

Exercises for arms and calisthenics can be classified into three different categories. Let's look each of them out.

- Biceps

These muscles extend out from the upper portion of your arms. The below exercises to strengthen them.

Chin ups

Step 1: Find an adjustable bar that can withstand your weight.

Step 2: Attach yourself with the barre and utilize your bicep muscles to lift yourself slowly both up and down.

Step 3: Continue to do 15 lifts , then have a rest of 2 minutes before doing another set. Perform three sets.

Incline chin ups

Step 1: Sit in a position on your floor under the bar.

Step 2. Grab the bar using a firm grip , keeping your body straight from your head all way down to your feet.

3. Pull your back until the point where your chest is touching the bar, then slowly move down. Repeat the exercise 10 times.

Take a break for 2 minutes, after that, you can do 2 sets.

Korean dips

Step 1. Sit in the middle of the straight bar with your arms are securely holding the bar.

Step 2: Perform an extended down position in which your legs are placed under the bar and stretch them backwards.

Step 3: Lower yourself to your elbows in a 90-degree position. Utilize your arms to raise you back to your original position. Repeat this 10 times without taking a break. Take a two-minute break before doing another set.

To increase your biceps strength, try to build a routine that is effective for you. It is possible to aim for: 10 diamond push ups 10 chin-ups, 10 Korean dips 20 incline chin ups 10-dips in a straight bar 8 negative chin-ups, and lastly 10 dips.

- Triceps

These muscles protrude below your arms. Exercises for triceps include:

Bench dips

Step 1: Sit on a bench and place your hands on the bench and allow your body to hang up with the help by your arms.

Step 2. Your body should be parallel towards the bench. The next step is to lower yourself till your elbows sit 90 degrees.

Step 3. Utilize your arms to lift yourself up back to the starting position. repeat the exercise 15 times, then rest and complete two sets.

Push ups for the triceps

Step 1: Lay on the floor with your back to the ceiling.

Step 2: Put your hands on the floor and bring your arms close to your chest. Then gradually pull yourself up then back down using the triceps muscles.

Step 3: Repeat the exercise 20 times more

Wall push-ups

Step 1. Step 1: Stand in the wall in front of it with your feet about at a distance of four feet from the wall.

Step 2: Set both hands against the wall, with your palms only a few inches from one another.

Step 3: Lower your chest to the point that your nose is touching the wall. Then use your arms to pull yourself up to your original position. Repeat this exercise 20 times.

- Forearms

The forearms of your forearms play an vital role in helping support your body while you're performing some of the calisthenics exercises. Let's take a look at some exercises you can try that will strengthen the forearms.

Supported hangs

Step 1: Hold on to the bar using your hands, then raise yourself and hang from there. Your legs shouldn't be touching the ground.

Step 2: Stay to this position until exhausted. Recover and repeat the workout 10 more times.

One arm hangs

Step 1: Find an incredibly strong bar that will support your weight and then attach it to the bar using one arm.

Step 2: Remain in for this posture until exhausted. Repeat the exercise 15 times.

Shoulders

Training with body weights strengthens the shoulders significant way , but you'll be required to warm up prior to doing the exercises. Push-ups and arm circles are excellent examples of warming exercises you can perform. Here are some calisthenics exercises that will strengthen your shoulders.

Exercises for beginner

Modified push-ups

Step 1. Find a spot in which you can lie down, then elevate your body to an upward position by using your hands and knees.

Step 2: Slowly lift yourself up and then down. Repeat 15 times, take a break and do another exercise.

Pull up the plank

Step 1: Lay down and then get into an upright position.

Step 2. Lift yourself up in the same manner as you would in a push-up, but instead of falling you should hold your highest point for a few seconds.

Step 3: Repeat this workout until you're exhausted.

Advanced exercise

Handstand with one arm supported

It takes time to master, so don't be in a the rush to complete it. Do it slowly and you'll soon be able to do it.

Step 1: Place yourself against an exterior wall. Then, bring to you a bench to rest your arm free.

Step 2: Lift your body to form the shape of a handstand with two arms.

Step 3. Find your balance using the two-arm handstand , then gently lift one arm off the floor and place your hand on the table to provide assistance.

Step 4: Stay in at this point until exhausted, then switch arms, and repeat the exercise for a few sets.

Chapter 15: Training for Weight vs. Weight Training Using Bodyweight Which Is Right For You?

As you read this book, you're attracted to bodyweight training. However, let's first examine the benefits of weight training and bodyweight training and determine which one you prefer over the other. While I'm not saying that, I am a fan of bodyweight training but I also enjoy weight training too. I believe that each is beneficial in the training process. I do recommend weight-training for my clients based on their needs, and do suggest bodyweight training in addition.

Here are some pros and cons for each method of training.

Pros of weight training

Progressive overload is simpler to do, where you simply take heavier weights, and put the more hefty weight to the bar.

* It's easier to understand the motion of the exercise. You are able to master a few compound movements and other exercises can be performed using the machine and do require the learning process.

Cons of weight training

* Attach a shearing press (most dangerous pressure) onto your joint hindering your endurance of training.

* You must purchase an exercise membership or pay for equipment

Pros of bodyweight exercise

* You can perform this exercise wherever you want! Think about doing these exercise before taking off your shirt to display the hard work you've put into it!

* It doesn't cause too much stress joints because the pressures applied to your joints is not shearing pressure but rather direct pressure.

Training with bodyweights can be a disadvantage

The process of progressive overload can be a a bit more challenging because to get the proper amount of progressive overload you have to introduce a variety of exercise choices rather than adding weight.

* Always discover new types of exercise.

Review this list of pros and cons and choose which one you prefer to be focusing on. You are free to select both methods because I implement both methods for my clients regularly.

This is the time to answer this issue with you. Are you convinced that you can be jacked by weight training? I am talking Arnold Schwarzenegger Jacked. Think about it for a second... It's no and yes. By training with bodyweights, you could attain that body shape of Arnold Schwarzenegger However, the proportion of your body may not be as exact as Arnold. This is because bodyweight training is heavily focused on the concept of COMPOUND MOVEMENT.

Compound movement is that involves more than one piece of your muscle is used to lift the weight. These exercises do not concentrate on your muscles, such as the calves, biceps and biceps. If you're looking to build calves and biceps that pop, I would suggest that you incorporate weight training along with your bodyweight exercise or leave bodyweight training altogether and instead do exercises that require weights.

Chapter 16: Advanced Calisthenics

Advanced Calisthenics

If you've been working out in calisthenics over the past few months, or you're an athlete who is advanced and looking for an exercise routine that is new There are certain to be some difficult and efficient exercises you can do.

Advanced calisthenics can provide the amazing benefits of building a strong muscles, while also creating higher levels of intensity. Be prepared to sweat more to breathe harder, and increase the endurance of your muscles.

Different kinds of Advanced Calisthenics Exercises

You can create a program that incorporates a range of calisthenics exercises. Certain advanced exercises force your body to utilize muscles you don't normally utilize in conventional exercise routines. With circuit training, you'll make the most effective workout with exercises in calisthenics that will help your body get in shape.

Circuit training follows the same idea as High Intensity Interval Training which is also known as HIIT. It is possible to combine the elements of cardio and weight training in one workout. It takes about 30 minutes to complete an exercise routine for calisthenics is more efficient than slaving for 2 hours in an exercise facility.

For each of these exercises, do at minimum one set of each of these exercises without time between sets. Each exercise should be completed in 30 second intervals. The intense exercise will surely increase your heart rate up, and your muscles forming quickly.

JUMP SQUATS

Be tall and straight, and make sure you spread your weight evenly across your heels.

Lower your body to the squat position. Your arms should be extended behind your back.

In a frenzied movement Jump to the highest height you are able when you lift your body out of the squat position.

Make use of your calf muscles, then raise your arms above your head. Make sure you maintain your straight legs when you are going up.

When you are landing, gently put your feet on your feet, then lower to a squat.

Repeat the steps for throughout your remaining time.

HANDSTAND

Place your feet spread shoulder-width apart. Make sure that you have plenty of room surrounding you.

Bring your body forward and place your hands on the floor while you stretch your legs straight towards the sky.

You can support your body by using the strength of your shoulders. Keep your core active and pay attention to your breathing.

Keep this position for 30 seconds.

After you have come down then bring your feet towards the floor and bend your knees in a way that you return to your beginning position.

SINGLE-ARM PUSH-UP

Put yourself into the position of a push-up by placing one of your hands on the floor and your feet large.

Engage all of your body and put your free hand against your back.

Slowly lower your body towards the floor. Bend your elbow slightly as you descend.

With your single arm, bring it back up to the original position. Make sure you keep your muscles healthy.

Do about 10 reps, then change arms.

Repeat steps until you've completed through 30 seconds of the workout.

JUMPING LUNGE

Keep your height up and keep your feet stumbling. Keep your knees supple and slightly bent, but don't keep them fully extending your legs.

Maintain your core in place and then jump off your feet and switch directions of your feet up in the air.

Relax your body in a classic lunge. Make sure to straighten down and keep your front leg thigh in line with the floor.

Repeat this exercise, alternating between legs.

Repeat this sequence for 30 seconds.

These sophisticated exercises, when combined with the HIIT circuit training program will help you build incredible muscle mass and give you an enviable bodybuilder shape you've always wanted.

Chapter 17: Engagement, and Goal Setting:

The most impressive thing about calisthenics working out is its total independence! You can train any time, anywhere, and with an array of different movements and routines. What's not to love?

It's awe-inspiring when you understand what you're doing, but if you're brand new to this type of workout or any other exercise, this could lead you to be confused. Particularly for newbies it is essential to have a plan of action that is well-thought out to establish an effective foundation.

Establish your goals:

Objectives are a crucial part of calisthenics.

It is essential to be aware of your goals including weight loss and power improvement as well as the increase of muscles, enhancing general fitness and endurance and achieving the ability to carry out a precise job out, such as an exercise that is known as the "human flag. Diverse goals require different approaches. It is vital to figure clear what you want to accomplish, due to the reason that different goals require different strategies in the way you exercise.

What should I do to start?

This is a big subject!

It's a good thing! Much like everything else in life, you must start with the basics before having fun by doing difficult exercises like front lever, planche , and human flags.

Take a walk on the floor to do a few push-ups. Simple isn't it?

Don't look for more efficient methods as it takes an amount of time to transform your body into a muscle. But, it's essential for you to set goals in a brief amount of time so that you stay active. Instead of making it a brief deadline, push your self to create it an integral part of life! In addition, you need to excel at the little things like:

Diverse pull-ups workout is vital to strengthen your v-shape, upper limbs and upper limbs. It also helps strengthen subordinate muscles such as your abdominal muscles, as well as your shoulders.

PushupsThis workout will build your strong chest and triceps muscles as well as subordinate muscles such as your shoulders.

Squats: This workout is designed to strengthen your legs.

Diverse dips activity will help build the whole body above the waist.

Abdominal exercises: They are designed to provide you with a solid central muscles that is vital for calisthenics.

Leg raises: This is the perfect exercise for those who have not been working the lower abdominal muscles, as well as the hip flexors (the muscles of the iliopsoas.)

Regularly performing leg raises will give you the lower back, and thus reduce the chance of injuries.

Every complex and difficult move is just an alteration or mishmash of the fundamental exercises. You must therefore be a steady performer in those basic composite exercises so as to build up strength within your body.

How can you progress in calisthenics effectively? :

There are a lot of guidelines for development that you should know. In the end you can get any skill gained by becoming familiar with these ethical principles.

DECONSTRUCTION

It is simply about dedicating an extensive amount of your time to study the art of doing it from beginning to the end. When it comes to calisthenics you'll have to practice the posture of the hollow body. This is intended to strengthen the muscles that are your primary strength. the best thing to do is to do the following exercises to a great extent:

Intense squatting

Dead lifting

Kettle bells

Swings and grabs

Sandbag squats

Shouldering

If you aren't willing to add weights in your exercise routine, there's the possibility that you will be in a position to create an impressive lower back. In any case, you must be focused on concave body positions bridges, handstands, and handstands.

CONTINUAL CONFRONTATION: Keep learning and enduring as an established habit. Try to push yourself with increasing the difficulty continuously. Although it might not be that easy, by attempting it repeatedly, you will improve your skills in this.

STEADINESS:

According to American soccer coach as well as player Vince Lombardi, "Practice does not always make perfect. Only practice that is perfect makes perfect."

So you see! There is no quick way to master the art of hard work, hard-earned practice and perseverance; it's claimed that in order to excel in anything, you must put in at least ten thousand hours to run through. Actually it's not enough to just need some time to practice, but an extensive and consistent practice. The ability to tolerate and be steady are the key to positive results for you. Even if you've got knowledgeable knowledge about the field and are doing the best job but without consistent efforts, it's just speculation. A few guidelines to help you stay on track are:

Set reasonable goals which include clear highlights, and as you progress towards your goals, you'll notice the ripple effect and things start to become more logical in your daily work, household routine, and your physical condition.

Set a consistent workout time in your calendar. This is the standard practice that has been endorsed by the most dedicated fitness enthusiasts; the majority of them do every day prior to sunrise or at night.

If you're looking to be more authentic with your body, you should take an additional initiative on your calendar for the day and try to dedicate 30 minutes each day. As a result you'll have more energy and will be more organized. In the end, you'll be able to are more energetic and be more productive during the course of your day. It is also possible to utilize cell phone applications, like emails on a day by day basis. exercise tracker websites, and apps that help keep you focused.

Keep a daily journal to track your progress It will not only motivate you to work harder, but also help you in deciding which steps in the right direction.

Track your progress by keeping track of each tiny achievement. The goals you set for yourself regarding what you'd like to achieve within the next few months, are simple to track Each small achievement can help you stay motivated.

Keep a record of your thoughts following each calisthenics exercise in order that when you're in a slump of energy to wake up and get active then you can take it off and look back at the thoughts written down by you after you have completed the calisthenics exercise with success. This will make you realize that in the end of the exercise, you'll feel the same sensation.

Try a miniscule exercises on a regular basis in order to help you maintain your regimen of exercises throughout the week. Miniscule workouts can comprise of core exercises, regular push-ups, and hang-ups.)Your core functions as a counterbalance, hub and counter. This means that when the actual training sessions begin and you will be training, only a small portion of your effort will be put into.

Chapter 18: The Perfect Execution

Don't think about being a winner. Work hard for it.

Without going too far into the realm of science and going into the technical details we'll take a look at what flawless execution is in the context of Calisthenics. It's a brand new way of workout that you're only getting familiar with this, and we'd like to help you learn more about how to perform it right the first time. Here are some crucial aspects to be aware of.

Modifying Your Body Position

You can participate in what's known as "progressions" through simple workouts. When you do a push-up, for instance, you can perform it using your knees on the ground. You can gradually move up to no knees before moving on by elevating the feet over your head while doing the push-up.

When you move your muscles from the tuck to a straddle posture using push-ups, you will be able to exercise your muscles more vigorously. Then you begin to utilize the bones as levers and your joints act as fulcrums, with the muscles that are there to exert pressure. This shift can cause the center of mass away from the body to the shoulder by straightening your body. This may make it more difficult to apply torque to the shoulder, especially when you raise your feet, and so on.

Resting Length

Muscles are the strongest when they are at rest length. In this stage, greatest number of cross-bridges are created. A cross-bridge occurs when the contractile part that is part of the muscle, myosin as well as actin - meet in a way, where the myosin pulls against actin to tighten the muscle. If you cut or extend the muscles while you put a heavier load onto the body it could trigger an adaptation like if you were carrying the heavier weight.

Training Concepts

It's crucial to be aware of the following definitions before you start building out your calisthenics workout routine:

Repetitions: Sometimes reduced in reps. The amount of repetitions you can do in a single workout can determine the intensity of the exercise. Ten push-ups can be done in a row, before taking a break after completing one set.

Sets: The amount of reps you are able to do in a session is referred to as an "set. As many sets as you perform the more challenging a workout will become. It Is typical to perform 10 reps three times, in three sets.

Rests: This refers to the time that is taken to rest between activating the muscles. There are short periods of rest as well as long rest times.

Tempo: This refers to the time at which you complete your repetitions. It is commonplace during "high-intensity interval exercise" where the participant will try to complete as many repetitions of an exercise as quickly as is possible in 60 seconds.

Load: This refers to the intensity of your exercise; i.e. you could generate a greater load in Calisthenics by elevating your feet over the head's angle in a arm exercise.

Volume: The amount of exercises completed in a single exercise.

Understanding Repetition vs. Strength

There is a continuum of repetition that is present within the realm of Calisthenics. It indicates strength at one end, while endurance is at the other. The strength side can be achieved by a low number of repetitions and weights that are heavier, at slow paces. The endurance side involves lighter, by performing more repetitions or having an increased tempo. This is why you must know the following:

It is impossible to build strength and endurance with a single exercise. You must create the schedule to prioritize both.

The time you spend strengthening your muscles will increase your endurance and the reverse is true.

Strength requires more time to develop than endurance training for basic purposes.

Quality is not the same as. Quantity

Quality is always more important than quantity in Calisthenics. These are workouts which specifically engage various muscles, tendons and even your entire nervous system. This isn't about strength, massive weights or even showing off. It's about engaging the entire body in an efficient workout that's been practiced for hundreds of years.

So, take the notion that you need to do "number number of reps" from your head. Actually, a lot of times it is much more challenging if you complete only one repetition (a squat) and do it for 60 seconds.

As stated above the most effective way to build your strength is by engaging in isometric exercises. Reps that are performed in a steady and slow method, moving through your body at a high speed is the way you will achieve the greatest gains in the least time. Stop focusing on the number of reps in the fitness center.

Systemized Resting

Your body is an enthralling machine made up of hundreds of moving parts. If you exercise one of these moving parts (muscles during the day prior) it is possible to let them rest for on the following day when you focus on another group of muscle groups that were not stimulated during the workout.

We've mentioned this before and that is the reason you are now aware of all you must know about flawless execution in the realm of Calisthenics.

Chapter 19: How Can I Lose Weight By Calisthenics?

Yes, you can. Alexander describes it this way that the greater your muscle mass the greater the metabolic rate of the body. Therefore, you can shed weight with ease by performing calisthenics.

Where can I get calisthenics classes?

The greatest benefit of calisthenics is the ability to perform the exercise at any time, from anywhere . It can be done as

* Home exercise

* in nature, or

* at special calisthenics park.

The pull-up bar are not necessarily required. If you are doing a workout at home it is possible to do the calisthenics workouts without aids. If you're outdoors in nature, a tree can be utilized as a pull-up bar or you can make use of the playground to create a workout space.

Be cautious: Always ensure that you are not putting at risk yourself or other humans if you do not make use of aids like scaffolding or branches that are specifically made for training in calisthenics.

Exercises for Calisthenics for beginner

For those who are just beginning begin by practicing the basics of exercises until you're able to perform them correctly and in a controlled way. According to ALEXANDER fundamental exercises consist of :

* Pushup

* Squats

* Pull-ups

Also, work out gradually . This means you are able to complete an exercise without difficulties, or increase the difficulty by introducing a new variant (for instance, one-handed push-ups) as well as increase number of repetitions.

In this article we will go over the three exercises that are fundamental to your training in the previous article, as well as three additional exercises to help you begin your calisthenics workout.

3 calisthenics exercises with no training equipment

The following self-weight exercises to get calisthenics at home.

Basic exercise such as push-ups

* Difficulty level Medium

* Target muscles: pectoralis major

* Muscles supporting: triceps anterior deltoid muscles, cartilaginous muscles anterior saw muscles

Place your knees on the floor and your feet on the ground less than shoulder width apart front of you. The hands must be approximately an inch above your chest. Stretch your legs and step on the tip of your toes. Reduce your body with control until your nose is almost touching the floor. You can then push yourself back up.

Be sure that your torso, head and legs remain in straight lines. Additionally the arms shouldn't be straightened in order to ensure your joints are protected. If you're looking to safeguard your wrists, you can utilize special handles to do push-ups.

In the next video, Timo explains to you how to perform the correct push-up and how to utilize the handles.

Tips for women who are just beginning Women's

Push-ups if you don't have sufficient strength to do push-ups, sit your knees down to the ground and then bend your legs a bit.

When you wear the women's push-up, you reduce the weight on your arms, which means it is much easier.

Squats are the most basic exercise.

* Level of difficulty Easy

* Target muscles : quadriceps, hamstrings, gluteal muscles

* Supporting muscles Back extensor, three-headed adductor

Standing upright, your feet shoulder-width apart. Move your arms horizontally forward. Slowly lower your buttocks down and extend to your knee joints till your knees are level with the floor. Keep the position for a few seconds and then lift up your back and push upwards. Be sure your knees are in line with your ankles.

In the next video, Timo explains how to complete the squat properly.

Planks

* Difficulty level medium

* Muscles: all body muscles, including the back, trunk, leg hip and gluteal muscles, as well the chest and shoulder muscles.

display

Set your forearms down on the floor, parallel to your body, and then put your elbows underneath your shoulders. You can place down your hands on the ground or lock them. Like push-ups. The entire body should create straight lines. You should hold the position for approximately 1 minute or for as much as you can.

In the next video, Raoul shows you which errors to avoid when making plans and how to strengthen the posture of your plank.

3 calisthenics exercises using training equipment

In order to perform the exercises, you'll require the equipment for training that is typical of calisthenics

* Chin-up bar

* Ingot or dip bar

1. Basic exercise The basic exercise is pull-ups

* Difficulty level Medium

* Training device : (pull-up) bar, branch

* Target muscles: broad back muscle lower fibers of hood muscle, the large and small rhomboid muscles large round muscle

Back extensors arms flexors, biceps Upper arm spoke muscles

Lean on the bar using both arms and lift your body until your chin touches the bar. Slowly lower your body back to the bar.

In the video below, Timo explains exactly how the proper way to pull-up is performed:

For beginners, learn how to pull-up

You can't do a pull-up yet? Not a problem, the following steps will allow you to master your first pull

Exercise 1: Hold on to the bar for as long as you are able to.

Second exercise: Your shoulders should be lifted up slowly, so that you lower and raise your shoulders a little.

Third exercise: Place an exercise band on the bar, sit on one leg or with your knee inside the band, and perform your first pull-ups while supported.

Exercise 4: Perform horizontal pull-ups. This could be done on a bar, or under the table in the kitchen.

2. Dips

* Difficulty level Medium

* Training device : dip bar or parallel bars

* Target muscles are triceps cartilaginous muscle anterior part of the deltoid, pectoralis Major

• Supporting muscles short and long extensors of the hand radial hands, ulnar hand extensors common finger extensors and little extensors of the fingers

Utilize using the grip that is neutral to get yourself up onto the bars. Don't raise your elbows up to safeguard your joints. Then you can train your chest or work your triceps muscles:

1. Chest

Keep your chin in your chest, extend your legs inwards and move your upper body forward. Begin to lower yourself slowly and with a controlled movement until your arms are level with the floor. The elbows shift towards the side.

2.

Keep your triceps straight as you look ahead and extend to straighten your legs. When you lower yourself with control make sure your elbows are in close proximity to the body. The bottom of your downward motion is at the point that your angle of lower and upper arms are 90 degrees.

Joe explains how you can do proper dips by watching the next video.

3.Hanging leg raises

* Difficulty level Medium

* Training device : (pull-up) bar

* Target muscles: straight abdominal muscle and muscles of the pyramidal

* Supporting muscles: oblique abdominal muscle

Secure the bar using both hands , and then raise your legs to a 45-degree angle. Lower your legs with a controlled movement. If you are strong in your abdominals, you are able to stretch your legs. Be sure to keep your legs in a straight line always.

In the next video, Johannes explains everything you must know about your Hanging Leg Raises:

Chapter 20: Equipments used in Calisthenics

The benefit of an exercise program like Calisthenics is that it requires almost no equipment needed to perform the exercises. All you need for the necessary equipment for a highly effective calisthenics workout can be found at any play or playground. You can find horizontal bars and dip bars monkey bars and many other equipments provided it's safe to use it. There are also fitness centers in a variety of nations that offer a variety of bar layouts, such as different heights and thicknesses. These aren't very well-known but you shouldn't need to be concerned if you do not live close to one of these locations.

It's not that you use only items to perform moves and actions on. Numerous books I've seen that deal with bodyweight exercises suggest that you use a variety of common household items in your workouts. There are a variety reasons, it's not a good idea. The first reason is the fact that the majority of household appliances aren't designed to perform pull-upsor dips and other exercises with them, in accordance with the weight of your body. If they fall or break during use there is a chance that you'll be injured.

Calisthenics also comes with the benefit of acquiring the equipment and equipment that you require would be simple. The material used to make the equipment made is usually affordable, easily available and not difficult to construct. This is in stark contrast to treadmills, friction plates, rowing machines, cross trainers as well as weight plates and Olympic bars and so on. They can be expensive to purchase and to maintain. You'll find there's it is not necessary to maintain dip or pull-up bars!

In the coming weeks in the coming weeks, we'll look at the different types of equipment used for calisthenics-related training on, where you can find it, and the importance of each component will be in your overall success.

THE LOCATION for training

The first thing you need to consider before you begin training for your Calisthenics is the location you will train in. It's a major choice because the most important factor is to take pleasure in your workout, since when you aren't able to locate a good spot and you don't like it, you're likely to quit. There are many places that are appropriate and I'll go through some of them below.

For calisthenics training fitness centers and gyms that are commercially owned are fantastic and anyone who reads this book is near one of these places. The benefits are that they typically contain plenty of equipment, they're in the indoors, which means the schedule of training won't get affected by the weather as well as the costs are reasonable. However, you'll be paying for a variety of facilities (such like swimming pools and so on.) that you won't receive a lot of value from. The type of equipment they have will not be a great fit to exercise. Cross Fit gyms are one type of exercise that's great for Calisthenics. No matter what you think and I have many regarding Cross Fit, it can be said with certainty that they've got some excellent facilities and equipment that is perfect for those who want to start doing Calisthenics.

The second option is playgrounds and play areas are alternative for those who wish to exercise using Calisthenics, but do not want to join the gym or invest any dollars on the equipment. Today, many playgrounds come with different pull-up bar and dip bars, as well as tables, monkey bars ropes, tables. They can be far more convenient to use than a gym that is commercially owned. The drawback is that nearly all parks and playgrounds are in the open, and If you're planning to use the area to train then you'll need to deal with the surroundings. If you're in an area that is dry and warm it's not a issue, but it's an issue to be considered. The other option is to protect yourself. Playgrounds are usually designed specifically for children. Problems with adults exercising near children could occur. It is recommended to talk to the local authority in this instance to determine whether it is suitable to exercise in the area. You could also hold off until the children went to school, and it would not be a problem.

The third option is to make use of an area specifically designed to be an area of training to train bodyweight and Calisthenics. If you reside within or around the U.S. or Eastern Europe or Russia these are getting more popular especially in cities which is where they will typically be found near or connected with basketball courts. They aren't as popular in England however, they are becoming more accessible because of initiatives to encourage youngsters. These kinds of fitness centers generally have a range of Bar thickness bars as well as dip bars parallels, etc. Another benefit of these types of places is that you will meet others who are eager to improve as you do and having learning partners and groups is among the most effective ways to progress.

The last location you have to train is inside your home. This may require purchasing or building some equipment and it's likely that you won't have a calisthenics facility that is already built in the home you purchase or relocate to. But, that does not mean that you have to spend a lot since the majority of the equipment needed for calisthenics instruction is cheap and easily accessible. In the next segment we'll take a take a look at a few tools used for calisthenics and bodyweight exercises and what they should include and where it is located, and alternative options to the items you buy.

THE PULL-UP BAR

Although equipment isn't necessary for Calisthenics exercises, performing every pull-up exercise without a pull-up bar is a challenge, possibly impossible. An exercise bar that can pull you up is the ideal piece of equipment to do that. It's not only possible for use a pull-up bar for any pulling exercise however, it can be utilized for a variety of routine exercises, as well as some pushing exercises. This could make it the most affordable piece of fitness equipment ever developed. The gyms in both locations must be equipped with these devices and if they do not then don't go in or change gyms. If the gym doesn't possess this essential piece of equipment needed to perform Calisthenics then I'm afraid to imagine what else they do not have. If you're lucky you'll find bars that aren't right next to the ceiling, which will allow you to perform the muscle-ups quickly. If you're not currently an active gym member however and don't have any plans to join one, there's various options for those who are.

You can purchase one pull-up bar in the beginning. If you choose to follow this route and follow it, it'll be one of the most beneficial options you have in your fitness journey. There are many different types of pull-up bars that range from ones that attach to walls and others that can be inserted into door frames, and are even stand on their own. You can choose one that is flexible to fit your needs and budget. I have the PowerBar in my home and have utilized regularly for several years. It has never failed me and was extremely affordable and will fit a variety in door frame styles.

If you're not able to afford an adjustable panel or you're able to put one anywhere, there are plenty of options. One of them is to use any object over your head that can be grabbed. This could include the stairs that are below the basement or basement, a balcony or even a limb of trees. As long as the thing that you are attempting to use it on can support your weight in a safe manner, then I can see no reason pulling exercises can't be done on it.

DIP BARS

Dip bars are another popular piece of equipment that is found not just in gymnasiums that are commercially owned but as well in play parks and training spaces outside. They are typically utilized for triceps dips like they are named, however, they could also be utilized to perform a variety of exercises, such as levers that go back and front as well as muscle-ups, handstands as well as planche. Dip bars in commercial gyms are usually linked to larger pieces of equipment, like leg raise and pull-up bar stations. They aren't ideal for calisthenics-only workouts in certain instances, but they are still a great option. Dip bars are significantly longer at playparks, meaning that three or four people can be exercising simultaneously, or ride in them, change direction to do handstands, planks and more. You'll have a great exercise. Dip bars are available in a variety of varieties, with various bar widths, thicknesses, and heights, similar to pull-up bars. It's difficult to find stand-alone dip bars that you can purchase however, if you search online you may find some.

Since I've got the space in my home, I've built a set of dip bars in my back garden, and if you have space and the spare time, I strongly encourage you to do that as well (as long as the wife/husband/partner/parents of course allow). By building your own, you can alter the size to fit your body type and shape and build the bar as long or thin as you'd like. If you're thinking of building your own, an immediate Google search will bring up numerous tutorials on how you can do this.

PARALLETS

In a few ways they are similar to dip bars in the sense that they comprise two bars that are separated distance, but facing each other. Parallets differ in that they are usually smaller and higher than the ground. If you've looked at bars for push-ups, then parallets are like larger models. They can be utilized to power movements such as handstands, push-ups, planche work, and more. The benefit is that you are able to broaden and reduce the grip size since they are distinct units that fit your specific body. They can even be taken virtually everywhere since they are extremely compact and easy to carry. This is a great option for those who travel frequently or travel for business or don't have the space to create a space for training at home.

Parallets are available in a variety of kinds, but there is several items to consider when purchasing they:

The reason is that they need to be durable. The reasons for this are evident. If you're doing the handstand position it is important to not allow the handstand you're making use of to malfunction, as it is likely that you will harm your self and others.

Second, they require a bar that's easy to grasp. Parallets with dimensions of less than less than a couple of inches isn't ideal, and while it can be beneficial to the strength of your grip, it could make it more difficult to manage handstands, boards, as well as other workouts. There are plenty of sites where you can purchase online parallels, so it's a good idea to take a look for what discover.

* Like I mentioned, the third option is to build your own. It's a simple process and plenty of money could be saved. There are a variety of instructional videos and tutorials out available that can instruct you on how to build fitness equipment online such as parallels. Searching for parallels will result in a quantity of results, but in my own research, the fundamental structure is evident as an image. will be shown below.

As it appears, one piece of dowel that was around 30 millimeters in diameter and cut it half way. Then I set up small pieces of wood until there were four, that were 10-12 inches high. Then, they were screwed and the dowel ends were attached onto the towers. It's clear that they are handmade, but I've owned these for around five years, and they've always impressed me.

It's crucial to ensure that you set the right spacing between parallets. It will be different to each person, but the most efficient method is to place them in a space that is shoulders wide. This will ensure that your hands are just below your shoulders while doing handstands, planks, half levers, etc. This makes your life easier since your arms will act like columns in the vertical direction that are able to support the rest of the weight of your body. You could either stare into a mirror and see the length that your shoulders are, or engage a partner in training to assist you. If you aren't able to do that the width of your shoulder will generally be about the same as the distance between the tip of your fingers to your elbow. Just make sure you align your comparisons using this equation and you'll be fine.

Conclusion

For a final note It is crucial to keep in mind that while you do the exercises mentioned above, in case keep eating processed and unhealthy food items do not expect any loss of weight or body shaping. Therefore, there is the need to follow an enlightened diet, as we mentioned earlier. Additionally, you need to stick with it: consistency can pay dividends.

www.ingramcontent.com/pod-product-compliance
Lightning Source LLC
Chambersburg PA
CBHW060333030426
42336CB00011B/1317